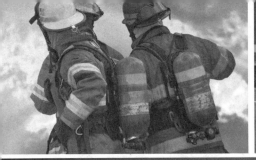
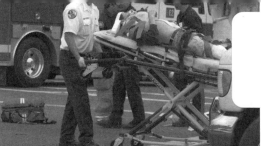

CREW RESOURCE MANAGEMENT

PRINCIPLES AND PRACTICE

Paul LeSage, FF, EMT-P, AS, BA, CFM
Jeff T. Dyar, NREMT-P, BS
Bruce Evans, MPA

JONES AND BARTLETT PUBLISHERS
Sudbury, Massachusetts
BOSTON   TORONTO   LONDON   SINGAPORE

World Headquarters
Jones and Bartlett Publishers
40 Tall Pine Drive
Sudbury, MA 01776
978-443-5000
info@jbpub.com
www.jbpub.com

Jones and Bartlett's books and products are available through most bookstores and online booksellers. To contact Jones and Bartlett Publishers directly, call 800-832-0034, fax 978-443-8000, or visit our website, www.jbpub.com.

Substantial discounts on bulk quantities of Jones and Bartlett's publications are available to corporations, professional associations, and other qualified organizations. For details and specific discount information, contact the special sales department at Jones and Bartlett via the above contact information or send an email to specialsales@jbpub.com.

Production Credits
Chief Executive Officer: Clayton Jones
Chief Operating Officer: Don W. Jones, Jr.
President, Higher Education and Professional Publishing: Robert W. Holland, Jr.
V.P., Design and Production: Anne Spencer
V.P., Manufacturing and Inventory Control: Therese Connell
Publisher—Public Safety Group: Kimberly Brophy
Senior Acquisitions Editor—Fire: William Larkin
Associate Editor: Laura Burns
Associate Production Editor: Sarah Bayle
Associate Photo Researcher: Jessica Elias
Director of Sales: Matthew Maniscalco
Director of Marketing: Alisha Weisman
Marketing Manager—Fire: Brian Rooney
Cover Design: Kristin E. Parker
Cover Image: © Crystal Craig/Dreamstime.com; © Lisa F. Young/Dreamstime.com; © Les Cunliffe/Dreamstime.com; © Michael Ledray/Shutterstock, Inc.
Composition: diacriTech
Text Printing and Binding: Edwards Brothers Malloy
Cover Printing: Edwards Brothers Malloy

Copyright © 2011 by Jones and Bartlett Publishers, LLC, an Ascend Learning Company

All rights reserved. No part of the material protected by this copyright may be reproduced or utilized in any form, electronic or mechanical, including photocopying, recording, or by any information storage and retrieval system, without written permission from the copyright owner.

Some images in this book feature models. These models do not necessarily endorse, represent, or participate in the activities represented in the images.

Notice: Unless otherwise noted, the individuals described in Case Studies throughout this text are fictitious.

Additional photographic and illustration credits appear on page 156, which constitutes a continuation of the copyright page.

Library of Congress Cataloging-in-Publication Data
LeSage, Paul.
 Crew resource management: principles and practice / Paul LeSage, Jeff T. Dyar, Bruce Evans.—1st ed.
  p. cm.
 Includes index.
 ISBN-13: 978-0-7637-7178-2
 ISBN-10: 0-7637-7178-3
 1. Emergency medical services—Management. I. Dyar, Jeff T. II. Evans, Bruce E. III. Title.
 RA645.5.L47 2009
 362.18068—dc22
                      2009028580
6048
Printed in the United States of America
19 18 17 16 15   10 9 8 7 6 5

Brief Contents

CHAPTER 1 Introduction 1

CHAPTER 2 Organizational Story and Culture 8

CHAPTER 3 Creating a Culture for Learning 22

CHAPTER 4 The Critical Decision Process 37

CHAPTER 5 The Concepts of Crew Resource Management 47

CHAPTER 6 Understanding and Implementing Crew Resource Management 71

CHAPTER 7 Leaders, Followers, and Teamwork 92

CHAPTER 8 Postincident Analysis 113

CHAPTER 9 Maintaining High Reliability 127

References and Resources 147

Glossary 149

Index 152

Photo Credits 156

Contents

CHAPTER 1 Introduction 1
    Introduction 2
    By the Numbers..................... 2
    Humanware 3
    Preparing for CRM................. 5
    Summary 5

CHAPTER 2 Organizational Story and Culture 8
    The Power of Story 10
        How Cognitive Dissonance Affects Our Story 12
    Mining Stories to Change Organizational Culture 14
    Managing the Story: Changing the Culture 17
    Writing Our Own Story.............. 18
    Summary 20

CHAPTER 3 Creating a Culture for Learning ... 22
    A Stronger Foundation for CRM: Establishing a Just Culture 25
    Placing Blame 25
    What Is a Just Culture?............... 26
        What is Accountability?.......... 26
    Complacency Kills.................. 27
        Deviations from Protocol......... 27
    Establishing and Losing Trust 28
        The Right Reaction: Taking Responsibility 30
        Postincident Analysis 30
        Sytemic Cause Analysis.......... 31
    An Important Piece: Self-Reporting and Trend Files................... 32
    A Summary of a System Failure 32
    Why Develop a Learning Culture?...... 33
    Summary 34

CHAPTER 4 The Critical Decision Process..... 37
    Understanding a Complex Process 39
    The Role of Conflict 39
    Event-Driven Scenarios and CRM 40
        Key Factors in Decision-Making Efforts 40
    Decision Process Risks and Rewards 42
    Summary 45

CHAPTER 5 The Concepts of Crew Resource Management 47
    Developing a Shared Understanding..... 49
    CRM: A Comprehensive Approach........ 50
        The Role of the Team Leader 51
    Building Team Expertise and Flexibility 54
    Removing Boundaries and Establishing Trust and Respect 54
    Choosing a Method of Engagement 57
    Team Behaviors: The Differences between Novices and Veterans 57
    Team Behaviors: Keys to Maintaining Situational Awareness 58
    Minimizing Factors That Cause Loss of Situational Awareness 62
    Improving Collective Situational Awareness by Understanding Error ... 65
    Reducing Distraction and Staying Focused 65
    Instituting Situational Awareness Within a Culture 67
    Summary 68

CHAPTER 6 Understanding and Implementing Crew Resource Management 71
    Working with an Open Communication Model: The Circle of Success 73
    Inquiry........................... 74
        Factors Affecting Inquiry: Coherence and Sense Making ... 74
    Advocacy......................... 76
        PACE.......................... 78

Conflict Resolution 82
Decision. 83
Observe and Critique 85
Discuss Options. 87
Summary 88

CHAPTER 7 Leaders, Followers, and Teamwork 92
Leaders: Envisioning Goals and Setting Clear Objectives. 94
Delegating Authority, Taking Responsibility, and Gaining Commitment. 95
    Delegating Authority. 95
    Taking Responsibility. 95
    Gaining Commitment. 96
The Leader's Ability to Maintain a Dynamic Situational Assessment 96
Understanding Individual and Team Limitations 97
The Ability to Adjust 98
Valuing Team Diversity 100
Listening Aggressively and with Curiosity. 100
Mentoring 101
Relationship Management for Leaders. . 102
Effective Followers 103
    Challenging Decisions as an Effective Follower. 105
    Getting to Know the Team Leader 107
    Lifelong Learners. 107
    Types of Follower Behavior 107
Poisonous Team Member Behaviors. . . . 108
Summary 110

CHAPTER 8 Postincident Analysis. 113
Motivations for Postincident Analysis 115
Assumptions behind Postincident Analysis 116
Tailboard Debriefings. 116
Types of Incidents that Warrant a PIA 118
Techniques for Conducting a Formal PIA 118
Tools for PIAs 119
Idiosyncrasies of PIA. 124
Summary 124

CHAPTER 9 Maintaining High Reliability 127
Introduction to High-Reliability Organizations 129
Develop a Habit of Mindfulness. 129
Avoid Mindlessness. 132
Assess the Ability to Inquire, Doubt, and Update 133
    The Ability to Inquire. 133
    The Ability to Doubt. 134
    The Ability to Update. 134
Become Preoccupied with Failure 136
Be Reluctant to Simplify 138
Be Sensitive to Operations 141
Commit to Resilience 142
Defer to Expertise. 142
Summary 143

References and Resources 147
Glossary 149
Index 152
Photo Credits 156

Chapter Resources

Crew Resource Management (CRM) enables public safety teams to make the right decisions in the field quickly, safely, and together. CRM stresses the importance of having strong leadership in place to guide a team's decision-making process, while encouraging individual team members to share critical information to help the team leader make the right decisions during an emergency.

Crew Resource Management: Principles and Practice shows emergency response leaders how to implement CRM skills in their fire stations, in their ambulances, in their police vehicles, and on the emergency scene. The key features of this program include:

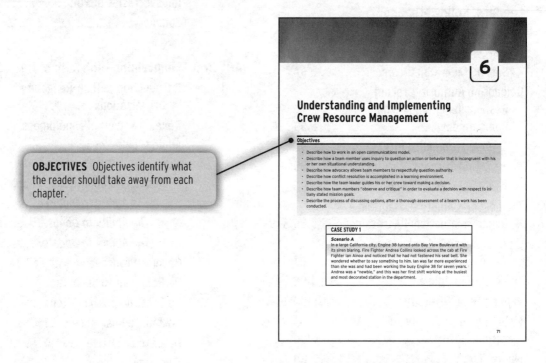

OBJECTIVES Objectives identify what the reader should take away from each chapter.

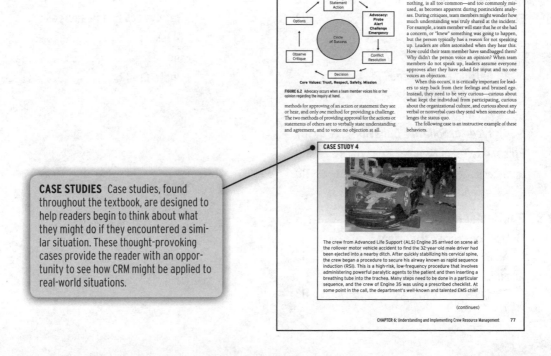

CASE STUDIES Case studies, found throughout the textbook, are designed to help readers begin to think about what they might do if they encountered a similar situation. These thought-provoking cases provide the reader with an opportunity to see how CRM might be applied to real-world situations.

READY FOR REVIEW Ready for Review highlights critical information from the chapter in a bulleted format.

ASSESSMENT IN ACTION Assessment in Action study questions are provided at the conclusion of each chapter to help readers apply what they have learned. Answers can be found in the Instructor's ToolKit.

VITAL VOCABULARY Key terms and definitions are highlighted throughout the text. A complete list of each chapter's terms and definitions appears in the Wrap Up section at the end of that chapter.

REFERENCES References are provided by the authors as suggested further reading on CRM implementation. A complete list of these references appears in the back of the book.

IN-CLASSROOM ACTIVITY In-Classroom Activity appears at the end of each chapter, as a resource to guide instructors through the introduction of key CRM concepts to students.

Instructor Resources

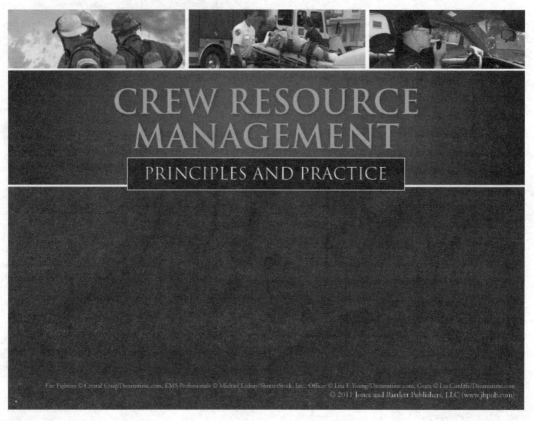

Instructor's ToolKit Online
ISBN: 978-0-7637-8370-9
- *PowerPoint® Presentations* correspond with the book and can easily be personalized to suit each instructor's teaching style.
- *Lecture Outlines* provide a format for instruction and align with each of the PowerPoint slides.

To purchase access to the Instructor's ToolKit visit www.jbpub.com.

Acknowledgments

Jones and Bartlett Publishers would like to thank the following individuals for their review of the manuscript:

Gary L. Aleshire, Jr.
Assistant Fire Chief, Shohomish County Fire District #1
Everett, Washington

Bill Betts
Fire Officer II
Commissioner, Delaware State Fire Prevention
Milford, Delaware

Jim Critchley
Assistant Chief, Tucson Fire Department
Tucson, Arizona

Scott D. Glowaski
Deputy Chief, Shohomish County Fire District #1
Everett, Washington

Larry J. Grorud
Fire Chief, Janesville Fire Department
Janesville, Wisconsin

Jon Holcombe, MPA, EFO, CFO MIFireE
Fire Chief, Hamilton Township Fire District #2
Mercer County, New Jersey

Jeffrey D. Johnson
Fire Chief, Tualatin Valley Fire & Rescue
Tigard, Oregon

BJ Jungmann
Public Safety Instructor, Century College
White Bear Lake, Minnesota

William Walton
Chief, Delaware State Fire School
Dover, Delaware

Author Biographies

Paul LeSage, FF, EMT-P, AS, BA, CFM

Assistant Chief Paul LeSage works for Tualatin Valley Fire and Rescue, an agency serving over 430,000 people in the Portland, Oregon Metro Region (www.tvfr.com). He has over 30 years of experience as a fire fighter, paramedic, flight paramedic, command officer, and educator, and has degrees in Organizational Communications and Sciences. He is on the faculty at Oregon Health Sciences University as a Clinical Assistant Professor and lectures nationally in the emerging fields of Fire and EMS Crew Resource Management, Critical Decision Making, High Reliability, and Deployment. Paul also built a publishing business from the ground up, and has authored several Fire and EMS Field Guides, along with articles and book chapters related to deployment and decision making.

Jeff T. Dyar, NREMT-P, BS

Jeff Dyar began his career in the fire service in Brighton, Colorado in 1971 as a volunteer EMT. Since then, he has worked in private, public, academic, military, and federal capacities and has authored four books. Mr. Dyar held the position of Program Chair for EMS, Firefighter Health and Safety, and Counter-terrorism at the National Fire Academy in Emmitsburg, Maryland for 12 years. Jeff has worked at some of the largest events in modern history, assisting local response agencies on behalf of FEMA and the U.S. Fire Administration, including both World Trade Center events, 18 hurricanes, the Columbine School shooting, and the 2002 Winter Olympics. Jeff was the Chief of Operations for National Emergency Operation Center for FEMA and oversaw dozens of national events. He was recognized by the White House in two administrations for outstanding service and is a recipient of the James O. Page Award for his national contribution to Fire Service EMS by the International Association of Fire Chiefs. Jeff currently resides in southern Colorado and serves as a Fire Commissioner and President of the Board for the Upper Pine Fire Protection District in Bayfield, Colorado.

Bruce Evans, MPA

Bruce Evans is the Assistant Chief of Business and Support Services at the North Las Vegas Fire Department in southern Nevada. Mr. Evans is an NFPA Fire Instructor III and coordinates the College of Southern Nevada's Fire Technology programs, teaching various fire and EMS topics. Bruce has over 25 years of experience in a variety of EMS settings and is an adjunct faculty member of the National Fire Academy in the EMS, Incident Management, and Terrorism Training programs. He is the Chair of the National Association of EMTs' Safety Committee and was appointed to the Safety Subcommittee of NHTSA's National EMS Advisory Committee. He holds a Master's degree in Public Administration, a Bachelor's degree in Education, and an Associate's degree in Fire Management. Bruce is a member of the IAFC EMS Section and a certified faculty member for the International Public Safety Leadership and Ethics training program. Mr. Evans writes the bimonthly column, "EMS Viewpoints," in *Fire Chief Magazine* and is on the editorial board of the *Journal of Emergency Medical Services*. He is also a board member for the Cyanide Treatment Coalition and coordinates the James O. Page Mentorship Program.

Prologue

Many words have been written regarding how individuals can communicate more effectively. In the best of circumstances, when two people have a discussion, there is time for them to develop their thoughts, clarify statements, and actively listen to one another. Even then, miscommunications occur. Unseen barriers that affect understanding between two individuals include personal context, perceived or actual hierarchical difference, cultural disparities, life and work experience, personal and organizational motivations, and a host of other factors. (See **FIGURE P.1**.)

In team environments, the opportunities for misunderstandings grow significantly. Typically, a team is a group of individuals who are brought together to achieve some sort of common objective. A high-performance team is committed to achieving the objective and holds its members collectively responsible for success, whether their individual skills are complementary or widely diverse. High-performance teams, by definition, require high-performance members, individuals who have proven to their organizations that they have the necessary knowledge, skills, abilities, and professionalism to handle difficult and complex scenarios. High-performance teams, however, suffer from the same types of communication failures as any other group, but because they are often composed of individuals with technical expertise, they can involve strong personalities and be difficult to lead.

What happens, then, if further complicating factors are added, such as severe time pressure, personal danger, loud noise, multiple distractions, or a confusing and dynamically changing environment?

Even high-performance teams that have proved their effectiveness in calm situations can find themselves frustrated and making dangerous decisions when they are faced with difficult and distracting environments. More importantly, organizational culture factors often contribute to the team environment, and individual members may fail to speak up during periods of high stress. In many instances, the team fails to achieve its objective because of ineffective communication, and in worst-case scenarios, people are injured or killed. (See **FIGURE P.2**.)

For example, in December 1978, on a very cold and clear evening in Portland, Oregon, the crew of United Airlines Flight 173, a fully loaded DC-8, found themselves flying in wide circles around the metropolitan area while they tried to resolve a problem with their landing gear. Less than one hour after discovering the gear problem, the aircraft contacted Portland International Airport with the following message: "Portland Tower, United One Seven Three heavy, Mayday. We're—the engines are flaming out. We're going down. We're not going to be able to make the airport." This was the final transmission from Flight 173 prior to the aircraft colliding with trees and homes in a populated section of Portland about 6 nautical miles (11,112 km) southeast of the airport. There was no postcrash fire because there

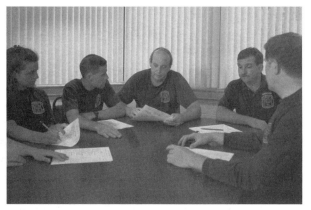

FIGURE P.1 Effective communication is the key to crew resource management.

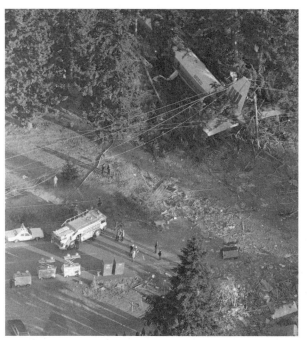

FIGURE P.2 Difficult and dynamic environments can contribute to dangerous, and deadly, decisions.

was no fuel on board—the cause of the crash was fuel starvation. Essentially, the plane ran out of fuel as the crew attempted to resolve the gear problem.

Miraculously, only 10 of the 189 people on board the aircraft were killed. The postaccident report listed causal factors that centered on poor collective situational awareness, failures in team communication, and misunderstandings related to the fuel system. In response to the accident, the airlines instituted a program in 1980 titled Cockpit (or Crew) Resource Management (CRM). Over the ensuing years, CRM training became a mainstay of airline safety programs. More recently, CRM-style programs have been introduced into other high-performance team environments, such as emergency medicine, fire fighting, and technical rescue/law enforcement.

There are many different methods for instituting CRM programs and specific safety objectives can vary widely based on the professional application; CRM can best be described as a method for enabling high-performance teams to achieve and maintain collective situational awareness. This is accomplished through a communication model that allows all members to communicate openly, respectfully, and honestly to manage errors, threats, distractions, and workload effectively. A successful CRM program also includes cross-training, planning, development of contingencies, and mission debriefing.

CRM is designed to break down the typical barriers to team communication, particularly those that have arisen over years of developing an organizational culture. Every organization has its hierarchy, its stories, its stars and experts. Every organization also has novice players, people with lots of experience but little rank, and those who are great at processing information but poor at verbally communicating.

The foundation of CRM rests on the collective power of the team. Rather than a "collection" of people, a "collective" is more powerful, where all team members form a whole, a single unit designed to work at maximum efficiency and using all the instincts and knowledge of every individual member (see **FIGURE P.3**). This collective relies on a communication model that is simple, elegant, and easy to follow. Although the model is simple, however, many organizational and individual barriers need to be overcome before it can be used effectively and reliably.

The CRM model assumes that team members understand their individual responsibilities and also that they recognize their important role as part of a unit or high-performance team that is assigned a task, a series of tasks, or an objective. In high-risk environments, all team members also have the knowledge that their domain can be very dynamic, and although the path to achieving their

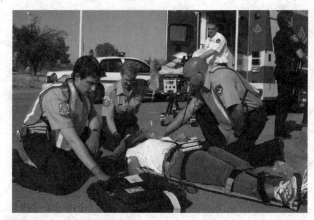

FIGURE P.3 When team members work as a "collective," they function as a single unit designed to work at maximum efficiency.

objective may be uncomplicated and undemanding when performed under normal circumstances, severe conditions or an accumulation of small errors can completely transform the original mission.

The first step in the CRM model of communication is recognition that a communication has been "sent" by a team member to be "received" by another. Recognition is the first step because it can be very difficult to detect specific types of communication and their relative importance during periods of heavy team activity, when personal danger is present, or when there are distractions. Additionally, these communications may take one of several different forms. They may be in the form of a statement ("I'm going to start an intravenous line"), a question ("Have you ever dealt with a fire involving fuel oil?"), an order ("Advance a line up the stairs to the second floor"), an observation ("It looks like the seizure activity is getting worse"), or a specific action or behavior. In many CRM models, this communication phase is called the *inquiry*. Inquiries take many forms, including those that are silent, such as body language or actions. For team members and team leaders, recognizing these cues while in the heat of the moment is a practiced art. Teaching team members how to see, hear, and prioritize these cues requires an interactive training environment infused with distraction.

Once the communication is received, regardless of its form, the receiver must either accept the message in its entirety or respectfully query to get clarification, gain understanding, or object. This phase, commonly called *advocacy*, requires probing (asking questions to clarify intent), alerting ("warning" the sender of the message about specific concerns), and challenging the message (a stronger form of alerting that typically dictates the team stop what they are doing until there is clarification and a decision by the leader).

Interestingly, an extremely high-risk behavior that commonly occurs during this phase of CRM (particularly in teams where intimidation or expert power are factors) is when team members say nothing at all, even when they see danger approaching. They allow verbal communications or behaviors to go unchallenged. In many cases, the team leader or other team members assume that the lack of input equals agreement. This is a specific danger for teams that operate with hierarchical assignments and titles. The following chapters of this book explore techniques designed to enable team members to understand the importance of speaking out and how to do so respectfully.

If the advocacy phase includes any type of alerting or challenging, the next phase of CRM is *conflict resolution*, in which team members resolve conflict during periods when they are engaged in critical thinking and the exploration of alternatives. This is a particularly important skill for the team leader to master and also requires "followership" skills from team members. All team members must be able to express their concerns diplomatically while at the same time determining which issues are mission critical and which can be compromised.

Once conflict is understood and resolved (even temporarily), a *decision* must be made. If the original strategy, behavior, or order is deemed appropriate for the situation and the skill sets of the team, the leader can decide to move forward. If, during conflict resolution, an alternative is developed, the leader can decide to engage the alternative strategy and monitor the outcome. Importantly, CRM is not team decision making. Teams have a designated leader for a reason, and organizations place individuals in positions of authority so that someone is responsible for making decisions. If not team decision making, the concept, then, is again best described as collective situational awareness: All members are aware of the objective, they understand each other's skill sets, they have voiced any concerns and vetted alternatives, and they move forward as a single unit, as a collective of people with a more complete awareness and understanding of the risks involved.

When the team leader makes a decision, the team continues to *observe* the effect of their actions and provide ongoing professional and technical *critique*. This critique process is typically demonstrated in a group through additional forms of communication that lead to statements, clarifying questions, observations, and actions. From these, options or alternatives can develop that lead back to the inquiry phase, after which there is more probing and alerting, followed by conflict resolution, and then yet again more decision making. It is clear how the circle of open communication continues in a manner that is

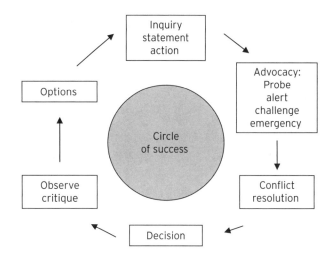

Core values: Trust, Respect, Safety, Mission
FIGURE P.4 The circle of success.

designed to make all members wholly aware of the situation. (See **FIGURE P.4**.)

A good CRM program demonstrates methods for clear communication within teams with an overall goal of ensuring that everyone involved understands the mission, the immediate goals, any dangers, and all known alternatives. Additionally, all team members should have a clear understanding of the risks that are associated with their actions or inactions.

Interestingly, it turns out that the simple and elegant model of CRM is not necessarily easy to implement in an organization. Embedded organizational culture related to positional status, "blame" environments, and a lack of understanding among policymakers about how to build resilient organizations are all factors that adversely affect implementing and successfully maintaining CRM programs.

Therefore, this book is not just about crew resource management. Primarily, it is about how we as individuals and as team members make decisions, particularly while under pressure. Cultural barriers associated with implementing an open communication process such as CRM are discussed, particularly within organizations that encounter dynamic environments and teams that are composed of domain experts, novices, and leaders with hierarchical rank. The dangers and acceptable errors associated with "trading accuracy for speed," which is a common problem medical, fire, military, and police operators face are also discussed.

To implement an open communication model such as CRM successfully, organizations must also address cultural and operational aspects that can cause CRM to wither and die, such as organizational story, the ability to capture mistakes and errors, and effective debriefings. This book also covers these critical issues.

Certainly, it is more difficult to change the culture of a large organization than a smaller one, Cultural change is made with small steps, however, through incremental movement toward an understanding of what is now considered "acceptable" behavior and what is not. Teams must build a strong cultural foundation in order for the framework of CRM to stand the test of time.

Finally, this book provides the tools to build a high-reliability organization that can understand the decision-making process, support mindful behavior, and embrace error as a method of learning.

Introduction

Objectives

- Define crew resource management.
- Describe how to achieve collective situational awareness.
- Describe the humanware component.

CASE STUDY 1

As the team from Engine 72 approached the front of the two-story apartment, probationary Fire Fighter Gano Yui observed heavy fire billowing out from the upper-story windows and smoke rolling from under the eaves. As he was taught to do in the academy, he paused to review the building construction and the primary routes of egress. His team leader, Lieutenant Scott Yost, gave the order to advance a hose line through the front door and up the stairs. Fire Fighter Yui was immediately concerned. He had observed a deformity in the roof line above the stairs and was curious whether his lieutenant or one of the other two veteran fire fighters on Engine 72 had seen the same thing. Fire Fighter Yui looked carefully at each team member to see if he could detect any traces of concern on their faces.

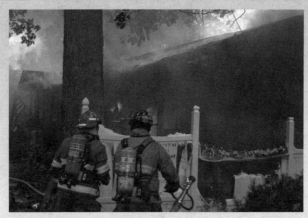

Lieutenant Yost repeated the order to advance and scanned the faces of his team. The two veterans nodded their approval. The four fire fighters made their way up the stairs and into the burning apartment. As they opened their hose line, a large portion of the interior ceiling collapsed, forcing all four fire fighters to the floor. Lieutenant Yost, at the rear of his team on the line, found the three fire fighters in front of him under debris and worked to free them while calling for assistance. All were able to exit the building safely, with two suffering moderate traumatic and burn injuries.

In the postincident analysis, the team of Engine 72 was asked if they had any concerns associated with their "standard" approach to this "ordinary" fire. Probationary Fire Fighter Yui was the only person to respond affirmatively. He stated that he had a concern about the roof immediately after the lieutenant gave the order to proceed upstairs. However, he acknowledged that he said nothing to any member of his team, and he also stated that he clearly understood what they were going to do because his lieutenant had repeated the strategy twice.

Introduction

Why don't team members speak up when they perceive something differently from how a group of their peers do? What are the effects of a hierarchal system on team performance? How can barriers be broken down to achieve collective situational awareness during critical events? How do veterans operate and perceive their surroundings differently from how novices do? Most important, what are the internal cultural barriers that impede optimal team performance?

By the Numbers

These questions are asked after nearly every major incident where a bad outcome causes an investigation. In recent years, one of the strategies integrated into emergency service team performance has been crew resource management (CRM). First developed and implemented by commercial airlines, *CRM* has become a commonly used term, and many agencies and organizations (air medical, fire, police, and hospital) have attempted to implement programs that rely on CRM principles. Unfortunately, in a recent survey of 11 agencies that had previously received CRM training, it was found that only 3 were effectively using CRM after two years, and the remaining 8 had failed to maintain any momentum with their CRM programs. The main reasons given were a lack of commitment by the leadership, lack of follow-up training, and a failure to implement nonpunitive methods for dealing with accidents, errors, and members who spoke openly regarding their concerns. Additionally, a commitment to developing open communication and CRM costs an organization time, and time equals money. Agencies that commit verbally to establishing a CRM program but then fail to provide appropriate staff support and funding are setting the stage for failure.

The fire service in the United States continues to experience an average of 100 line-of-duty deaths and more than 100,000 lost time injuries per year. A **line-of-duty death** is defined as a fatality to an emergency worker that occurs during the course of responding to, training for, or providing service to the pubilc. None of these deaths or injuries is considered an intentional act, yet most are preventable, and many have a root cause that could have been countered by the principles of crew resource management. As firefighting tactics evolve, fire fighters are less likely to be killed and injured by flames, smoke, or heat. However, traumatic line-of-duty death reports continue to reveal the effects of poor communication, weak teamwork, and bravado as significant factors contributing to a failure on the scene of emergencies. Communication failures, poor decision making, lack of **situational awareness** (being aware of what is happening), poor **task allocation** (directing specific workers to engage in specific tasks), and leadership failures are listed as the contributing factors in far too many **National Institute for Occupational Safety and Health (NIOSH)** fire fighter line-of-duty death reports.

In emergency medical services (EMS), the errors made in patient care could be contained by the implementation of CRM techniques in the high-risk, low-frequency procedures conducted in the field, such as advanced airway procedures. The number of medications placed on EMS vehicles is also getting more attention and consideration. The U.S. Food and Drug Administration received approximately 20,000 reports of medication errors (prehospital and in-hospital) from 1992 through 2002. Because many medication errors aren't reported, this number is a significant underestimation. In one study, 1 in 30 pediatric patients experienced a medication or procedural error. (See **FIGURE 1.1**.) The principles of CRM can help prevent errors in patient care.

With the extremes of fire behavior in the **wildland/urban interface** (geographical location where populated areas border wildland areas), the value of CRM becomes even more evident. Even experienced Type I incident commanders are reporting fire conditions never seen before. For example, as the amount of ideal suitable property for building homes decreases, development spreads into the wildland interface and communities are built on steeper hills and with fewer routes of egress. The buildup of natural fuels, scant controlled mitigation of fire risks, and the characteristics of these communities have led to firestorm situations that require critical interagency cooperation and communication. CRM techniques can be used in such scenarios when confronting extreme fire behavior and with a new generation of young fire fighters to open communication among technical experts, old fire hands, and novices. CRM can be an effective tool for adapting to and overcoming a changing environment.

The aeromedical industry continues to be one of the most dangerous professions in the country. The recent rate of helicopter crashes is alarming, and although the cost-benefit ratio and medical necessity of medical evacuation by helicopter continue to be debated, safe practices within the industry should be universally accepted. For a long time now, industry safety experts, the Federal Aviation Administration (FAA), and air medical organizations have promoted CRM training for ground crews and aeromedical crews. Yet a recent survey of air medical pilots showed that a majority believe the largest barrier to safety is a lack of commitment by their administrators to provide ongoing training and education. Although it is difficult to determine which particular factors might contribute to these beliefs, the lack of an industry-wide risk analysis tool that can be used for communicating "go" and "no-go" decisions speaks for itself. Here the regular practice of CRM techniques can contribute to a safer environment where all team members are collectively aware of the risks before flying.

When the U.S. Coast Guard employed the principles of CRM in its air operations, crashes and accidents were reduced by 70 percent. (See **FIGURE 1.2**.) Whereas some look for technology to solve problems, safety is clearly a human issue that can be affected by cultural change, error trapping, and ensured high reliability.

Humanware

When groups of competent, trained individuals get together to solve problems, they typically define the issue and then deploy a combination of "humanware," software, and hardware, to solve the problem. (See **FIGURE 1.3**.) In this context, "software" implementation can be rewriting training manuals or operating guidelines, or developing checklists, policies, and procedures. "Hardware" solutions can take the form of building construction modifications or the use of computers, vehicles, tools, medications, or protective equipment. The **humanware** component are

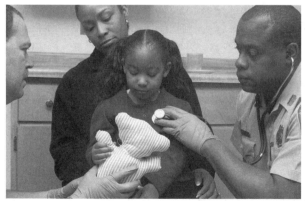

FIGURE 1.1 As many as 1 in every 30 pediatric patients experiences a medication or procedural error.

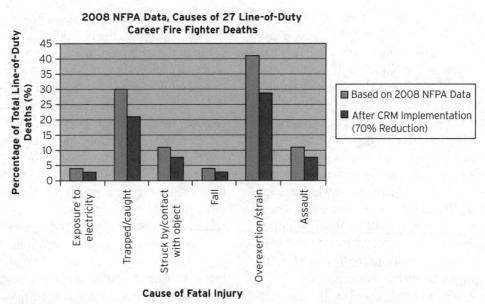

FIGURE 1.2 Implementation of CRM principles brought about a 70% reduction in line-of-duty deaths and injuries for the U.S. Coast Guard. A hypothetical example of CRM's potential effects is illustrated here.

Source: Adapted from NFPA, Fire Analysis and Research Division, *Fire Fighter Fatalities in the U.S.*, July 2009.

those people who are part of a team that has been directed to solve a particular problem (not the people who define the problem and provide logistical support). Open communication cultures that embrace respectful and informed feedback as a method for facilitating collective situational awareness develop skills for their humanware to solve complex problems effectively within dynamic environments. Essentially, they build communication skills and culturally ingrain them into practice.

Simply embracing an open communication environment and encouraging collaboration doesn't address all the human behavior aspects of organizational cultures and the differences in individual behavior and communication styles. An experienced and seasoned operator who is part of a problem-solving team understands that she will make little progress, regardless of how robust the system, if her human team members are unable to communicate effectively.

Incident command system (ICS) is a management tool used by people involved in managing emergency incidents to help identify incident needs and priorities. By identifying roles and responsibilities, outlining clear lines of communication, limiting span of control, and providing methods for expanding the incident, a well-developed incident command system allows leaders and managers to deploy resources in a structured and objective manner. When viewed retrospectively, some incidents used an outstanding ICS structure, but the resource allocation, communication, and incident management were poor, in some cases leading to the serious injury or death of operational staff.

What CRM can provide is behavioral expectations for the humanware involved in the incident. Because CRM uses a specific model of seeking input, acknowledging communication, respectfully providing differing opinions, resolving conflict, and monitoring a decision, CRM can highlight the areas where team communication breaks down. In addition, by retrospectively analyzing incidents and looking for the moments when team communications became ineffective, an organization can design specific strategies for improvement.

Whereas someone trained in the **National Interagency Incident Management System (NIIMS)** can easily implement an incident command structure, operating within that structure as a team member can be more difficult. Most of the education and training surrounding NIIMS is related to setting up the structure and operating within its constraints, but little attention typically is paid to the interpersonal communication aspects of maintaining situational awareness. For example, when a Strike Team is operating in the field, it is often little more than a "box" deep within a larger organizational chart of deployed resources. Implementing the principles of CRM, which include open and respectful feedback and a focus on collective awareness of the larger situation, can provide a much safer environment in the field and will result in a greater understanding of the mission goals and objectives by team members.

Open communication tools such as CRM help get maximum, safe performance from all personnel. Achieving a synergistic level of situational awareness is only possible if all team members understand the mission, the dangers,

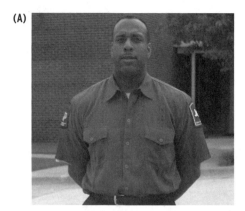
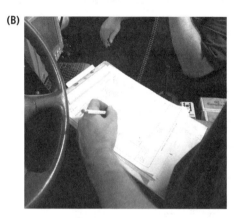
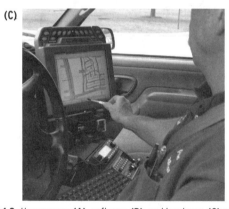

FIGURE 1.3 Humanware **(A)**, software **(B)**, and hardware **(C)** must be integrated for ideal results.

their strengths and weaknesses, and their role in team communications. Essentially, it matters little how well the organizational chart is developed if the people enacting the plan cannot communicate well with each other.

Preparing for CRM

Typically, when CRM concepts are introduced, they are embraced by all levels of the organization. CRM requires open and honest communication, immediate analysis of alternate probabilities, and a reliance on the strengths that each team member intrinsically brings to the team. These are seductive concepts, and they resonate with line personnel.

Once CRM has been adopted, however, the actual implementation is more difficult. Using CRM tools in an organizational culture that is not ready for open and honest communication at all levels leads to failure. Preparation includes training personnel in the techniques of open and respectful communication and developing a strong foundation so that the CRM principles will thrive. This foundation includes developing a comprehensive approach to identifying and tracking errors and mistakes, educating and training personnel in conflict management, teaching employees the power of organizational stories, and instituting regular and recurring critiques from which members can learn from each other. (See **FIGURE 1.4**.)

Summary

Over the next decade, approximately 1000 fire fighters will die and a million will be injured if the fire service continues down its current path. In addition, approximately 7000 people a year die from medical errors and more than 1.5 million people are injured as a result of medical errors. Emergency medicine has more technology and training than ever before, and yet errors continue to mount.

The answer may lie in creating a culture that accepts a certain amount of error within dynamic operations, separates operational mistakes from behavioral problems, and employs CRM-style open communication principles, thus promoting high reliability. If the fire service, EMS, public safety entities, and emergency medicine can adopt open communication models such as CRM and address the organizational culture issues that prevent learning from mistakes, the customer will be better served.

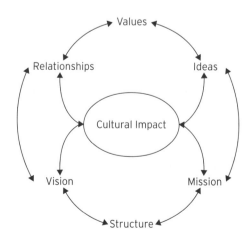

Dynamic Elements of Organizational Culture

FIGURE 1.4 The dynamic elements of CRM tools work together in an organizational culture to make a positive impact on the culture as a whole.

Wrap Up

Ready for Review

- Communication failures, poor decision making, lack of situational awareness, poor task allocation, and leadership failures are listed as the contributing factors in many NIOSH fire fighter line-of-duty death reports.
- CRM requires open and honest communication, immediate analysis of alternate probabilities, and a reliance on the strengths that each team member intrinsically brings to the team.
- Implementing the principles of CRM, which include open and respectful feedback and a focus on collective awareness of the larger situation, can provide a much safer environment in the field and will result in a greater understanding of the mission goals and objectives by team members.
- When groups of competent, trained individuals get together to solve problems, they typically define the issue and then deploy a combination of software, hardware, and humanware to resolve the problem.
- In EMS, the errors made in patient care could be contained by the implementation of CRM techniques in the high-risk, low-frequency procedures conducted in the field.
- An organization that has prepared its employees for CRM also has developed a strong foundation so that the CRM principles will thrive.

Vital Vocabulary

Humanware The people who are part of a team that has been directed to solve a particular problem.

Incident command system (ICS) A management tool that helps people manage emergency incidents by identifying incident needs and setting priorities.

Line-of-duty death A fatality to an emergency worker that occurs in the course of responding to, training for, or providing service to the public.

National Institute for Occupational Safety and Health (NIOSH) U.S. federal agency responsible for research and development on occupational safety and health issues.

National Interagency Incident Management System (NIIMS) A system used to coordinate emergency preparedness and incident management among various federal, state, and local agencies.

Situational awareness The state of being aware of what is happening to understand how information, events, and a person's actions will affect their goals and objectives, both now and in the near future.

Task allocation The process of directing specific workers to engage in specific tasks in numbers appropriate to the current situation.

Wildland/urban interface Geographical areas where populated areas border wildland areas.

Assessment in Action

1. True or False: In EMS, medication errors are frequently made because CRM principles are violated.
   A. True
   B. False
2. People who are engaged in problem solving are sometimes described as:
   A. software.
   B. hardware.
   C. humanware.
   D. work teams.
3. CRM techniques were originally developed by:
   A. the military.
   B. the airline industry.
   C. the fire service.
   D. law enforcement.
4. CRM requires which of the following elements?
   A. Seeking input
   B. Acknowledging communication
   C. Respectful communication
   D. Resolving conflict
   E. Monitoring a decision
   F. All of the above.

5. Which of the following elements is not part of situational awareness?
   A. Information
   B. Events
   C. Your own actions
   D. Maintenance logs

In-Classroom Activity

Review the scenario at the beginning of this chapter and conduct a classroom discussion about Fire Fighter Yui in regard to these situational awareness elements: on-scene information, building design and condition, tactics of interior attack, concerns of other team members.

2

Organizational Story and Culture

Objectives

- Describe the power of the story on organizational culture.
- Define organizational story.
- Define cognitive dissonance.
- Describe the effect of cognitive dissonance on organizational story.
- Describe how to use organizational stories to change the culture of the organization for the better.
- Describe how to manage organizational story.

CASE STUDY 1

Cadet Jeffrey Smith was excited about being hired by the fire department. One week into his class, he realized the rookie school resembled what he'd seen on television portrayals of the uniformed armed services. The yelling, belittling, and the retribution inflicted by instructors through intense physical activity until recruits vomited or collapsed created a culture of intimidation. Jeffrey believed this was normal. It was tradition; the entire training academy cadre, including the senior training officer, had been hazed while they were recruits. Over the course of several weeks, Jeffrey felt the tension mount. It became obvious that even little issues, "dumb" questions, and subjective uniform standards resulted in demerits and punishment, with instructors demanding that recruits perform an excessive number of push-ups or run until they were physically sick.

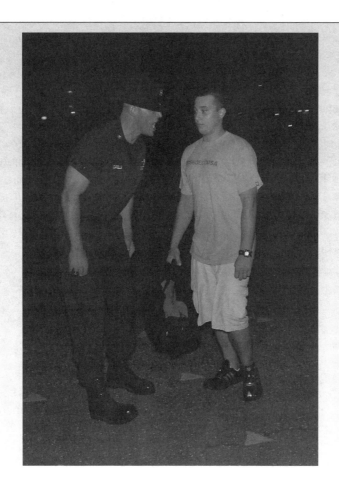

It became a culture of fear. Jeffrey learned not to speak up because the department culture rewarded those who stayed quiet during training and who didn't talk back or offer their opinions. On the first day of live-fire training, instructors set fires in an old abandoned house and the recruits were divided into teams and brought inside. As the heat continued to build until it was near flashover level, the instructors insisted the recruits stay inside to get some "real fire experience." Flames suddenly rolled across the ceiling and over the recruits, causing several to receive burns to their necks and body areas where their protective clothing was especially tight. As the recruits scrambled and rolled out of the structure, instructors pulled them together and told them they had now been "indoctrinated" into the fire service. "No one is injured, right?" asked the lead instructor. Jeffrey noticed that all the recruits looked around at each other, but no one said a word. The secret was theirs to keep, and he noted that the next day nothing was said about their experience. It appeared that all the significant safety issues that he had been taught to pay attention to had been ignored, and any reports written after the training fire covered up what had really happened. He did note that the following week, the recruits' activities were light to cover the injuries.

After graduation, the crew that Cadet Smith was assigned to continued to haze him. He was awakened in the middle of the night and made to "stand watch," criticized whenever he made a mistake, and was made to wear a t-shirt that said "Probie" across the back. The lack of sleep, belittling, and stress

(continues)

> reinforced the culture of fear that he had learned at the academy. At no time did Cadet Smith ever speak up, ask questions, or contribute to the crew discussions. Two months into probation, a working structure fire sent Cadet Smith and his crew to the roof of an older building to cut a ventilation hole. Cadet Smith observed a sag in the roof, and after stepping off the platform truck, he noticed the roof was extremely spongy and unstable. Because he "knew his place," Cadet Smith never spoke up, and within minutes his entire crew was scrambling for safety as the roof collapsed. Amazingly, no one is injured. After some half-hearted joking and laughter among the crew members, nothing further was said about their brush with death, and the crew returned to the station after the fire. Cadet Smith never mentioned the event, and he also never heard his officer or crew members discuss what lessons they may have learned from it. Cadet Smith left the department a year later.

The Power of Story

Nothing is more important to **organizational culture** than the stories that are associated with past events, personal behaviors, and future plans. Stories help people make sense of what they experience and create order in what they see, hear, and feel. Either consciously or unconsciously, people generate meaning through stories by shaping events into narratives. Narratives, the stories people tell themselves, become people's reality and help them define what to do and how to do it.

No program that is designed to improve team communication can succeed if people are afraid to speak up. Stories and how they are created can be used to introduce the open communication model of crew resource management (CRM). (See **FIGURE 2.1**.) Using a building as a metaphor, CRM is the framework of the structure, not the foundation. Although it's possible to build a framework without a foundation, the structure is unlikely to last long and certainly won't withstand any sort of "organizational storm." The foundation of any open communication model is the organizational culture, and that culture is built, and improved, by understanding how stories underpin "how we do it here" and "why we acted the way we did."

The rookie school experience should breed teamwork, not fear. Indoctrination into the fire service follows many good traditions, but hazing is not one of them. Hazing, bullying, and closing down avenues of communication introduce a culture of fear and intimidation. If the time is spent to teach new fire fighters the art and science of firefighting, it is expected that they will contribute their own knowledge to diversify and strengthen the team.

In Case Study 1, it is obvious that one **organizational story** at that particular fire department reinforces a culture of unprofessional and dangerous behavior. If allowed to continue unchallenged, bad behavior and bad stories become part of the organizational culture. Those who have been on the receiving end of hazing often believe the organizational "story" that it is okay to continue that behavior. Individuals who are taught through intimidation and through bad stories associate powerful narratives with what happens to those who speak up or who step outside the "norm" and report dangerous behavior. These team members remain silent, even if they know better, and even as they participate in actions that might lead to their own injury or death.

To understand how stories become embedded in organizational culture, it is important to realize that context is vitally important. When examining individual organizational stories, it becomes clear that many take the form of anecdotal comments that groups of people share when they get together to talk. Consider the story presented in Case Study 2.

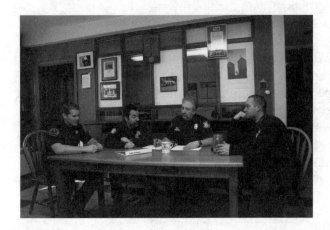

FIGURE 2.1 Use stories to introduce CRM.

CASE STUDY 2

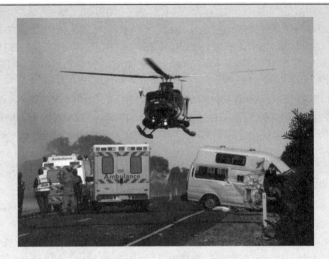

As the medical helicopter banks toward the Trauma Center, Flight Nurse Kim Davis adjusts the flow rate on the patient's intravenous (IV) line while simultaneously talking on the radio to the trauma physician. Flight Paramedic Pete Doyle, tired from the previous three flights, adjusts the monitors and prepares for landing. Winds buffet the aircraft, and he looks out the window and notes that the rain has started falling much harder since they departed the accident scene.

As the patient is off-loaded on the helipad, Pilot Howie Gregg signals to Kim by twirling his index finger in the air—they have been activated for yet another flight, an auto-pedestrian accident involving a child in a town 20 miles away.

Pete and Kim climb back on board as the twin turbines whine above their heads, the rotor slicing through the heavy rain mixed with snow that is now falling. As they lift off, Pete, sitting in the front of the aircraft with Howie, mentions to no one in particular that the "weather sure is starting to look nasty." Not getting any response, Pete sits silently until they are about halfway to their destination. At this point, Pete notices that the pilot apparently intends to fly direct, which will take them through a dark storm cloud and into instrument conditions, which is not allowed in their program. In his most respectful tone, Pete tells Howie, "I think we should turn around, the weather is getting bad."

Howie glances over at Pete and says, "Getting a little tired and cranky, are we?" At this point, Kim, who has been riding silently in the rear of the aircraft, pokes her head into the cockpit and says, "Pete, it's a kid. Same age as yours."

"Yeah, I know that," Pete says. "And I want to return to my family in one piece, so let's not break the rules here."

While Kim radios the scene that they will have to transport by ground, Howie silently turns the helicopter around. The ride back to the hospital base is a quiet one, even as Pete tries to stimulate some conversation.

Two weeks later, Pete is working with a different crew. As the pager goes off, he hears they are "tentatively activated, pending a weather check"

(continues)

> by the pilot. As Pete meets the pilot and nurse in the dispatch area, the pilot glances over and sarcastically says, "Well, I'm not sure my years of experience are adequate for this one. Let's have Pete the weatherman make the call." Pete is both embarrassed and intimidated. What have his peers been saying about him? Whatever happened to the open communication model, where no one was criticized for providing input?
>
> Although the weather is indeed marginal, Pete simply laughs off the comment and says nothing. The crew decides to launch. After returning to home base, Pete notes that they had flown through some very severe conditions, but feels he has no one to discuss his concerns with. The story is out there and can't be retracted. Pete's a chicken. He has made his last "team" comment during a flight.

How Cognitive Dissonance Affects Our Story

<u>Cognitive dissonance</u> is a state of mental tension that exists when a person simultaneously holds or hears ideas, attitudes, or beliefs that are psychologically inconsistent or contradictory. It produces mental discomfort that people feel a strong need to reduce, and it typically drives the need to self-justify and to develop or support narratives that are consistent with the person's beliefs.[1]

As an example, consider the many felony convictions that have recently been overturned because of newly available DNA evidence. In several cases, the original prosecutors vehemently deny making any mistake in the original prosecution. Regardless of the new physical evidence proving the defendant's innocence, the prosecutors maintain that the defendant "must" be guilty or he or she would never have been jailed in the first place.

Imagine you are a prosecutor. You spend your entire life doing the right thing—putting bad people behind bars and righting wrongs. You see yourself as a person who is thorough, meticulous, and just. You could never fabricate evidence to resolve a crime, and you know that you have released guilty people in the past for a lack of evidence.

Then, one of your previous convictions is questioned. It is a case you worked on for more than a year. You collected evidence, counseled victims, stayed up nights, and focused on developing the best case possible to win a conviction. You don't see yourself as a bad person, as someone who is careless, or as someone who could support an action that has kept an innocent person in jail for the past 20 years. Admitting you made a mistake in convicting an innocent person might lead to disgrace. Who would trust you after this? What if all your convictions come to be questioned? How do you right the wrong that occurred? How do you face a person who spent years in prison for a crime he or she did not commit?

These are examples of questions that might cause cognitive dissonance. A person's beliefs about him- or herself and his or her intentions and capabilities are powerful emotional anchors that often cause him or her to create excuses for what happened to deflect blame or to maintain a positive self-view. This tendency to shape or reinterpret information that doesn't "fit" with a person's view of him- or herself affects an individual's perceptions and the perceptions others have of their honesty and competence. More important, this tendency to relieve cognitive dissonance directly affects the organizational stories that people construct around certain events and can prevent them from learning. Consider the following case.

CASE STUDY 3

Ladder 7, driven by Apparatus Operator JR Jenkins and with a crew of three, pulled around the corner of Lexington Street and parked at the northwest corner of the Haney Auto Parts Store. Light brown smoke wafted from the front door, and Jenkins could also see some light smoke coming from where the front wall met the roof of the building. An experienced fire fighter in this town of 32,000, he knew the building well. It had been built in 1937 and was primarily brick construction with wooden roof beams that were supported on interior brick columns. He also knew that a drop ceiling, installed years ago, hid most of the roof support structure from view.

Before he could even exit the ladder truck, Battalion Chief C-102 ordered the crew of Ladder 7 to extend their main ladder up to the third-floor roof, and "Go have a look." Jenkins set the outriggers on the truck as his captain and fire fighter put on their self-contained breathing apparatus and grabbed some tools in preparation for their climb. Jenkins didn't like this particular ladder truck; it was a reserve, 20 years old, and the controls were known to be touchy. Within a few minutes, however, he had the ladder set up, with the tip hanging just over the front parapet wall of the parts store. The two members of Ladder 7 started their climb. As he reached the top, the captain called down that he wanted the ladder tip moved "a few feet to the left" so that he could step over the parapet and onto a short heating unit that was installed on the roof. Jenkins reached for the controls, and the ladder suddenly jerked hard left, spilling both the captain and the fire fighter over the edge of the ladder and onto the pavement, 36 ft (11 m) below.

The fire fighter, who lost his helmet on the way down and landed on his head, was killed instantly. The captain, a veteran of 19 years, critically injured his back and was retired from service.

A comprehensive external investigation found that the only possible cause of the accident was Jenkins bumping or moving the ladder control. There were no ladder controls at the ladder tip where the captain was, and an exhaustive analysis of the hydraulic and electrical systems proved everything was in working order. Although investigators did find that the ladder control on the turntable was "sensitive" to inputs, it was within the specifications posted by the manufacturer and by major standards-setting entities.

In the investigative report, however, it is apparent that Jenkins believes he did not touch the controls. In the first statements heard by witnesses, Jenkins is reported to have sworn and said, "Controls are so touchy the wind can move this thing." When asked directly whether he recalls moving the ladder, Jenkins states he not only didn't move the ladder, he wasn't standing behind the control box at the time of the accident. He repeated this story several different times, both to investigators and to other fire crews. During the postaccident interviews, investigators found several other fire fighters who repeated Jenkins's story. They had all seen him either on the turntable

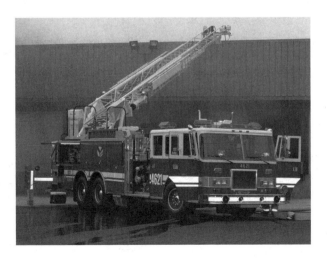

(continues)

> steps or at the base of the ladder; some even had him standing on the ground. None, however, saw him behind the control box. Even when video from a nearby convenience store confirmed that Jenkins was, indeed, standing behind the control box at the time of the accident, the story of him being elsewhere continued to perpetuate itself.
>
> The fire agency moved on. In the postincident analysis, no recommendations were made for additional training and awareness for the apparatus operators specific to ladder functions and behavior. Jenkins was not a liar, and neither did he mean to misdirect the efforts of investigators. Neither Jenkins nor his peers could "see" him making that grave of a mistake. The story that developed was more in line with the Jenkins they knew and was something he himself could live with. Unfortunately, the gaps left behind when cognitive dissonance drives a story often end up being traps that catch another employee unaware in the future.

Story is driven by a person's perceptions of events and by their inability sometimes to face what really occurred. CRM requires honest, open communication. It requires respect and an understanding of how each person provides value to the team. The moment a team member makes excuses for behavior instead of openly and frankly admitting an error, that team member has laid the foundation for an inaccurate story. This point is particularly important for the team leader to understand. If the team leader can diffuse the situation by acknowledging how errors are part of team learning, and if the leader can ensure that team members are treated with dignity and respect, the story that evolves from an incident typically is one based on the facts.

Therefore, when considering implementing a CRM program, it is important to understand how cognitive dissonance affects people and appreciate how it can affect organizational culture by obscuring truth.

Mining Stories to Change Organizational Culture

Stories combine motive, responsibility, and emotion. They provide a rich, understandable relationship between people, actions, and situations. In addition, as in the earlier story of Fire Fighter Cadet Smith, stories can affirm individuals' views of the organization and of themselves. When trying to persuade people, the strong appeal of a narrative story outweighs raw data or a dry set of facts. Stories are considered more "true" than raw facts because they weave the who, what, where, when, and how into an event. Stories involve personal relationships, moral issues, and conflict; they convey messages related to complex events while holding a listener's interest. This is important to know to understand how to change the organizational culture.

Within professional domains such as firefighting, emergency medical services, and emergency dispatching, no set of rules, regulations, or protocols can ever completely cover all the situations faced by industry professionals. "High-fidelity" training exercises, which are designed to be hands-on and introduce the **operator** (those on the front line in high-risk operations) to a dynamically changing situation with many variables, are becoming accepted as the finest form of preparation (see **FIGURE 2.2**). This doesn't, however, relegate books, manuals, and directives to the trash bin, but it does give some insight into how to work to change organizational culture from within, and how to make a culture more accepting of an open communication model such as CRM. Part of success lies in understanding the limitations of written policies and procedures, and how strict adherence to policies (even outdated ones) can affect organizational culture.

Although organizational guidelines, policies, and procedures can be written to handle some paradox and

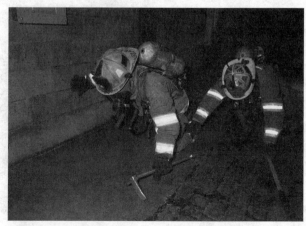

FIGURE 2.2 High-fidelity training has proven to provide the best environment for cognitive learning during complex events.

complexity, they are typically designed around what is known and specific "known unknowns"—those things that could happen but it's not clear how they might affect the team's operation. There are also "unknown unknowns." It is important to always be aware that "anything" could happen and to recognize that no one can write rules to cover every possible situation or variable.

In situations where the environment is dynamically changing, the rules known may not apply (or they are long forgotten). When a team must make quick decisions in which they trade accuracy for speed, it is proven that stories are what team members remember. Responders can recall a story they heard about how a peer faced a similar situation and succeeded or about how another individual's reputation was negatively affected because that person chose a particular course of action. Stories help in such situations because when stories are told they allow the listener to become involved in the dilemma facing the cast of characters, judge for themselves how the individual and team behaviors affected the outcome, and determine whether the organization's response was consistent and familiar with past history.

This is a helpful concept to grasp when trying to determine why a failure occurred or why an operator didn't act in accordance with written policy. People often try to "fit" the available policies to the situation, even if there were extenuating circumstances (or "unknown unknowns") that affect the team's behavior. One of the first things to ask after an incident is, "What story is connected to this event?" Operators usually appreciate an investigative approach that attempts to understand the motivating factors behind their actions, and they typically are more forthcoming in providing an accurate account of their behaviors and decisions. This is exactly the type of open communication that is necessary for CRM to thrive, but it requires an understanding that policies and procedures often take a back seat to organizational story. Consider the following in Case Study 4.

CASE STUDY 4

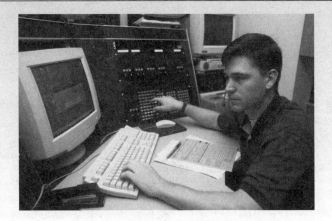

At the Monroe County 9-1-1 center, 46 dispatchers work the police, fire, and medical consoles every night on the graveyard shift. At any given time, four or five dispatchers are novices assigned to a veteran dispatcher who serves as their training supervisor. When Sandra Pujol called 9-1-1 on her cell phone at 2:31 AM, she was connected by the 9-1-1 call-taker to novice dispatcher Anna-Lee Bass. Listening in on another headset was Ed Karst, a veteran of seven years. As Sandra Pujol pleaded for help, the digital recording clearly picked up the sounds of breaking glass in the background while an intruder attempted to enter her apartment. Anna-Lee, shaken by the events, forgot to confirm the caller's address, which did not illuminate on the map in front of her because the call originated from a cell phone. In addition, Anna-Lee disconnected the caller after collecting the information and dispatching police.

Nine minutes passed before Sandra Pujol called 9-1-1 again to ask where the police cars were. The intruder was still outside, but was being held at bay only by her shouts that the police were coming. They were coming, weren't they, she asked? Moments later, the intruder entered the apartment, assaulted Sandra, and severely injured her.

The postincident review in Monroe County 9-1-1 center involved conducting a comprehensive systemic cause analysis. A **systemic cause analysis (SCA)** is a process in which every conceivable factor that could have affected the outcome is analyzed. After each factor is identified, a regression model is used to trace back every decision, equipment issue, training plan, or other influence that could have plausibly affected the outcome. (See **FIGURE 2.3**.)

In the case of Sandra Pujol, the SCA, among other things, noted that the training supervisor had the equipment, technical ability, authority, and responsibility to "barge" the call, that is, to take over for the novice when the trainee fails to perform. This procedure is outlined in policy and is covered in the trainee's course material, and the dispatch center provides the equipment necessary to ensure that the trainers are capable of barging when needed.

A simple resolution of this incident would have been to discipline the supervisor for not barging when policy said he should have. However, when it is desired to change the organizational culture and foster an environment where CRM techniques are used, further questions must be asked. Was Ed aware of the requirement to barge the call? Was he trained in how to do so? The answers to both questions are "yes." Had he done it recently? Had anyone? The answer to these questions is "no." As a matter of fact, because barged call recordings are kept for training purposes, it was discovered that no one had barged a call in more than four years.

Does this mean that in the period spanning those four years, no other dispatcher trainee at Monroe County 9-1-1 ever found themselves in a situation where a supervisor should have taken over? Of course not. In fact, when the SCA process dug deeper, the team members found that the last time barged calls were used for training purposes, a stigma was associated with those trainees who had their calls barged. The tapes were used over and over, voices were recognized, and a story was created that those on the tapes were somehow less professional and proficient than their peers were. In addition, the story developed to the extent where supervisors who barged were branded as overbearing and insensitive.

Over time, trainees became trainers, and they have long memories. The organizational story was that if someone barged a call, they stigmatized the trainee and were an overbearing and insensitive supervisor. Therefore, no one barged calls, regardless of what the policies said. Sandra Pujol, and by extension Ed Karst, were victims of an organizational story.

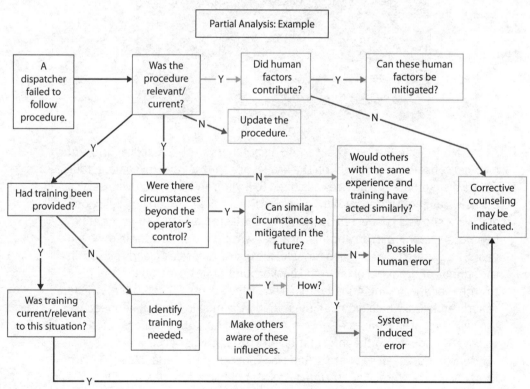

FIGURE 2.3 Although many different methods exist for carefully analyzing incidents, it is important to choose one that incorporates "just culture" practices. Any system that directs attention toward analyzing systemic issues, training, human factors, and environmental influence along with behavior is better than one that focuses solely on operator error.

In this particular case, it is an easy jump from "he didn't follow policy" to "he should be punished for it," and many organizations make that exact leap. Had punishing Ed been the resolution, the dispatch center never would have uncovered the true reason behind his behavior, and another operator would likely suffer the same fate in the future. Additionally, the result—punishment instead of curiosity—would have ensured that a strong stigma remained associated with speaking up during a critical event inside this particular dispatch center. Faulting error and ignoring organizational story are two of the most common causes that lead to failure of CRM programs. If the "foundation" is flawed, the structure hasn't a chance. In many cases, punishment or the threat of discipline can adversely affect attempts to create a collaborative, open communication environment that supports and promotes crew resource management.

Errors such as the one at Monroe County 9-1-1 need to be dealt with in the larger context of a learning organization, and individuals must not only take responsibility for their mistakes, they must learn from them. Simply acknowledging the error and moving on without individual and organizational learning is a shallow approach, and although it may put a good face on the problem, it will be perceived as less than sincere by the public. More important, by failing to capture the true causal factors of the incident, the organization avoids its true responsibility, which is to maintain the highest reliability possible during critical events.

Managing the Story: Changing the Culture

So, how can the organizational story be managed? Controlling stories within any organization is an impossible task, and attempts to keep people from talking about an event likely enrich the account with additional inaccuracies. There are, however, methods of helping those within an organization understand the impact of organizational stories and use them to mitigate damaging effects.

The first method of managing stories is to let all personnel know organizational expectations related to how they treat each other. Each person has the following responsibilities:
1. Operate with an open and curious mind.
2. Be respectful of team members and customers.
3. Communicate well.
4. Think before speaking (do you know the truth?).
5. Honestly admit weaknesses or mistakes.
6. Strive for high reliability through continual learning.

Next, examples can be used to emphasize the point and to demonstrate how individuals who mean well will not speak out if they fear the consequences of doing so. Their behavior, the failure to call attention to a potential problem, is often related to an organizational story. How was the last person treated when he or she spoke up? Were there obvious or subtle efforts to undermine the person's opinion, embarrass him or her, or diminish the person's standing with the team or organization? In such situations, regardless of training in open communication, implementation of CRM, and teamwork, few will dare speak up for fear of retribution.

In Chapter 1, Fire Fighter Yui neglected to speak up when his company officer proposed a plan of action. This story can be used as an opportunity to demonstrate another point about organizational story: People who perceive that they have less domain expertise or who are of lesser rank often remain quiet even when they hear or see something that disturbs them. No single individual can know everything, be experienced in all types of incidents, be calm and collected always, and be on top of their game every single day of their career—but it is still important for all to contribute their knowledge to the team.

Even after educating personnel and reminding them to pay attention to the risks of negative story, inaccurate narratives will circulate in the organization regarding individual or team behavior. An effective method for addressing these stories is to debunk them. **<u>Debunking</u>** a story is not denying that the event occurred. It is providing clarification, and also questioning the relevance of the story. This is easier if the story is related to a specific incident.

For example, see the earlier story about Flight Paramedic Pete Doyle. The story that started around Pete was that he was, essentially, a coward for turning around a flight in bad weather. This story is a good one to debunk. In this particular event, the facts speak for themselves: Pete did turn around a flight—that particular fact is accurate. The assumption made in the story is that at best, Pete is more risk averse than others are. This assumption can be used to direct a discussion on what the core values of the organization are. Debunking is also an opportunity to discuss how everyone has a different context from which they operate—what appears dangerous to one person may seem routine to another.

Leaders can debunk a story and set a new framework of expectations for individual behavior. By asking specific questions, the leader can help clarify for everyone what the expectations should be. For example, for Pete's flight program, the leader might identify which types of weather are to be avoided. If flying into instrument conditions is necessary, under what circumstances is it acceptable? Setting parameters helps everyone understand just how many individual viewpoints there are within the teams that form the flight program.

In the context of debunking, Pete can express what it meant to him to have his commitment to the program and to the patient questioned by others. He can use this opportunity to voice how the story impeded further discussion when he again found himself in poor weather situations; this degraded overall team situational awareness.

Another method of managing an organizational story is to provide counterexamples. Counterexamples rarely work on the first try. Instead, they are viral, like the original story itself, and require leaders to interject them when the leaders hear the "wrong" version of the story being told. Leaders should provide counterexamples that effectively disprove the original story. In Pete's case, leaders could tell two or three other stories of when Pete made difficult but accurate decisions. The counter stories may not even involve the flight agency; they might be about other people who failed to warn their team and suffered severe consequences. Like debunking, the use of counterexamples is most effective if the leader elects to pull everyone together and set baseline expectations for behavior.

Writing Our Own Story

Work environments where there is time compression (it is important to act fast), complex dynamics (the situation changes quickly and for reasons that are not always clear), cognitive challenges (a person faces something they have little experience with), and dangerous variables (failure to act can kill a person, their partner, or their patient) are challenging. Fire fighters, police officers, emergency nurses and physicians, and combat personnel commonly encounter these types of environments. In such situations, a person only has part of the information he or she wants in order to make a slower, more reasoned, and less intuitive decision. Once the situation is resolved, it is fairly easy to determine whether someone should have slowed down a bit and gathered more information before acting, or whether their quick yet less-than-perfect actions saved the day. Whether the trade-off of accuracy for speed was necessary often becomes vividly clear only after the event is over. Consider the example in Case Study 5.

CASE STUDY 5

As she pulled out from Grant Park, Police Officer Sandra Jamieson was flagged down by an elderly man who appeared to be out walking his dog. The man had just walked over the sidewalk on the east side of the Panorama Street Bridge, an early 1900s structure that spanned a deep canyon and joined two sections of the city's expensive upper west side. The local name for the structure was the "suicide bridge" because of the numerous people who had jumped from the span over the years. Signs on either end of the bridge sidewalk advertised the city's 24-hour suicide hotline.

The man had just observed a young woman in her early 20s climb over the bridge railing and sit on a small ledge below the level of the sidewalk. Officer Jamieson pulled her car alongside the railing, got out, and peered over the side. There, just 8 ft (2.4 m) below her, she saw a 22-year-old female on the concrete ledge with her legs dangling over the 340-ft (103.6-m) drop to the canyon floor. The woman would not answer any of Officer Jamieson's questions and appeared to ignore her entirely.

Eleven minutes later, Rescue 6 arrived with a crew of five fire fighters, led by Captain Neal Bodraw. Captain Bodraw looked over the side and immediately determined that his crew would don harnesses so that they could deploy over the side and pull the woman to safety. Officer Jamieson asked that fire crews stay back from the edge until a counselor could arrive who had expertise in talking with suicidal individuals. Captain Bodraw, stymied from allowing his crew to go over the rail, decided something had to be done, and fast, before the woman jumped.

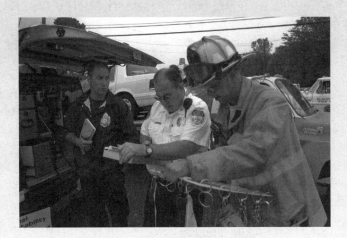

Without telling the police officer, Captain Bodraw and two of his crew members deployed over the west railing of the bridge, intending to climb through the lower infrastructure and emerge behind the suicidal woman. Because they were moving quickly and would be climbing on a steel structure, not hanging from ropes, the crew decided to forgo their normal practice of securing belay ropes to their harnesses from the road bed above. In addition, the captain said later, they felt that belay ropes would get caught in the lower infrastructure and "slow them down."

When Rescue 6's three-person crew moved past the approximate centerline of the bridge, one of the fire fighters slipped and fell 22 ft (6.7 m) to a lower beam, becoming wedged between two support posts that ended in a V shape. Had it not been for the posts, he likely would have rolled off the beam and fallen the entire 340 ft (103.6 m) to the bottom of the canyon.

The fire fighter's injuries were severe, and after a prolonged high-angle rescue effort he was transported to a Level One Trauma Center, where his left leg was amputated just above the knee.

In the meantime, Officer Jamieson talked the woman into climbing back onto the road, where she was taken to a psychiatric emergency center.

During a comprehensive postincident analysis, two of the crew members stated they were "uncomfortable" with the captain's tactics, yet they said nothing to him or to their peers. When the captain was asked why he employed such a risky strategy, he recalled a previous incident on the very same bridge five years earlier, when, according to him, "counselors talked the man to death—after three hours, he finally had enough and jumped while we watched, helpless to do anything." The captain was determined to act quickly so that the same thing wouldn't be repeated.

This is a classic case of trading accuracy for speed. However, note that it is the outcome that determines whether the trade-off was worthwhile. Had Captain Bodraw successfully come up behind the woman and secured her before she could jump, his actions would have reinforced that particular behavior as an appropriate tactic in similar circumstances.

Understanding and communicating the proper perspective to the workforce is a vital first step in helping them to appreciate that each person within the organization is "writing their own story" every time they face a situation in which they trade accuracy for speed. This will allow all employees to recognize that their own story is waiting to be told, and if they help to circulate an inaccurate story, they are contributing to a culture in which people criticize mistakes and errors, even those made during severe operating conditions.

If the outcome is positive, the story is generally good (Mary saved the day!). This can be because Mary is actually very talented and happened to be uniquely prepared to face the situation or because Mary was lucky. Either way, the story that is perpetuated reinforces the particular behaviors Mary engaged in when she faced that situation, regardless of whether they are consistent with organizational practice or policy. People will attempt to replicate the results next time in similar circumstances.

If the outcome is negative, the story is usually much different, even though there may be a perfectly reasonable explanation (Joe made a mistake). The systemic cause analysis may indicate that Joe's decision process, although it looks flawed in retrospect, was perfectly normal given the information he had at the time. What Joe can't control is the organizational story associated with the bad outcome. Despite the fact that Joe's actions may have actually been appropriate, the next time that particular situation is encountered, few people are likely to repeat his behavior. In addition, within many organizations, Joe would be stigmatized to a degree and his decision-making ability called into question the next time a similar situation arose.

Even more disturbing, stories like these cause people to associate specific attributes with individuals, and then they often look for patterns that confirm their bias. The fact that Joe performs flawlessly the next time can produce cognitive dissonance, and people may decide that based on his previous performance, he was just lucky this time. If Joe were to make another mistake, this would "confirm" the suspicion that Joe is inept, and the organizational story would be more firmly written and believed. Either way, if people don't confront their own tendency to build these stories, they won't likely be successful in breaking down the organizational tendency to simplify explanations and jump to conclusions.

Once personnel are educated about organizational stories, they can begin to understand that they could easily be the subject of the next story. Because they will begin to realize that their story will be "written" about actions and decisions they engaged in when they were pressed for time and information, they will be more obligated to question the veracity of narratives they hear in the future and less compelled to repeat stories that impugn the actions of others.

Summary

Maintaining an organizational culture that allows crew resource management techniques to thrive requires a deep look into how the organization manages its stories. Debunking and providing counterexamples are two ways to manage organizational stories. Regardless of how effective the CRM training is, CRM is only the framework of the open communication "building." CRM shows how the communication loop can work and how respectful, honest input can provide all team members with good collective situational awareness. The foundation of CRM is a good organizational culture, and a good culture understands the power of story.

Wrap Up

Ready for Review

- Organizational culture is heavily influenced by the stories associated with past events, personal behaviors, and future plans.
- Before implementing a CRM program, an organization must understand how cognitive dissonance affects people and appreciate how it can affect organizational culture by obscuring truth.
- Within professional domains such as firefighting, emergency medical services, and emergency dispatch, no set of rules, regulations, or protocols can ever completely cover all the situations faced by industry professionals.
- Regardless of how effective the CRM training is, CRM is only the framework that can promote open communication.

Vital Vocabulary

Cognitive dissonance The state of tension that exists when a person holds or hears ideas, attitudes, or beliefs that are psychologically inconsistent for that person.

Debunking The process of correcting information about events that have been inaccurately recorded.

Operators Those on the front line who are engaged in or in command of high-risk operations.

Organizational culture The psychology, attitudes, experiences, beliefs, and values (personal and cultural) of an organization.

Organizational story The texts, spoken or written, as well as visual recollections that usually involve a plot of different interconnected events and bind different characters together.

Systemic cause analysis (SCA) A class of problem-solving methods that intend to identify the systemic causes of problems or events.

Assessment in Action

1. Systemic cause analysis usually operates under which of the following assumptions?
   A. It is preventative in nature.
   B. It is a quality control measure.
   C. Emphasis is on punitive actions.
   D. It occurs after the event.
2. What is the position most likely to receive hazing in a dysfunctional department?
   A. Paramedic
   B. Rookie or probie
   C. Captain
   D. Training chief
3. Behaviors such as hazing have what effect on a crew of emergency responders?
   A. Positive team building
   B. Improved crew integrity
   C. Compromised communication and safety
   D. No real effects
4. Organizational story has what powerful effect on an organization?
   A. Heavily influences organizational culture
   B. Is usually an accurate portrayal of fact
   C. Never needs correction or debunking
   D. Is easily changed and controlled
5. An individual that is treated with respect and mentoring as a rookie will:
   A. not participate in open communication.
   B. not be relied on as a team member in a crisis.
   C. not respect authority.
   D. contribute to critical thinking in a team environment.

In-Classroom Activity

Lead a group discussion on the proper way to integrate a rookie into a functioning crew so that the rookie's introduction leads to crew integrity, effective communications, and acceptance by the other crew members.

References

1. Carol Tarvis and Elliot Aronson, *Mistakes Were Made, But Not by Me* (New York: Harcourt, 2007).

3

Creating a Culture for Learning

Objectives

- Describe how to create a just culture.
- Describe the practice of placing blame.
- Describe the danger of complacency.
- Describe how to reestablish trust with the public after a negative incident.
- Describe the role of self-reporting and trend files in creating a just culture.

CASE STUDY 1

As his partner Emergency Medical Technician Rhonda Miotta drove the ambulance deeper into High Springs Canyon, Paramedic Jon Morton slumped down in his seat, trying to get a few extra minutes of sleep. It was 11:30 PM on a hot summer night in the high desert country, and there was plenty of light cast by the full moon. Neither Jon nor Rhonda needed to look at a map to know where they were going; later court testimony would document that they had been to William Bidzil's residence 27 times in the past 90 days.

When the pager chirped 12 minutes ago and displayed the address, both Rhonda and Jon walked to the ambulance with a sense of resignation. Known as a "frequent flyer," Bidzil had a serious drinking problem and was well known in this small community. He was rarely transported to the hospital, was

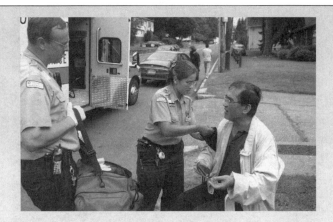

never violent with them, and usually wound up being taken by the ambulance or the police to the local detoxification center to sleep it off. Although the call usually came in as an "unconscious" person with trouble breathing, tonight was different. Jon and Rhonda had been dispatched to Bidzil's house on a "suspected snakebite." Because the occasional sight of a rattlesnake wasn't unusual in this rural desert community, it was certainly possible Bidzil or a family member had been bitten.

As they pulled up the long driveway to the house, Jon straightened up in his seat and noticed that William Bidzil was laying on the dirt at the base of the steps leading up to his porch. Surrounding him were his wife and three daughters. As Jon and Rhonda walked over with their medical equipment, he saw that Bidzil was sweating profusely and had multiple deep scratches on both arms. Bidzil was conscious, obviously intoxicated, had defecated on himself, and reported that he had been bitten by a large rattlesnake on his right arm and had subsequently fallen into a barbed wire fence while trying to run away.

EMT Rhonda Miotta, who had nine years of experience, all of them in this community, openly balked at the report. "I don't see any bites, William," she said. "I think you had a tangle with a fence, not a snake." Paramedic Jon Morton, out of school just three months, had never seen a snakebite. After carefully gloving up and putting on a paper gown to protect himself as he examined the feces-covered patient, Jon noted the deep scratches and saw that the bleeding was very minor. Bidzil's vital signs were relatively normal, other than a very rapid pulse. Jon turned to Rhonda and told her that he was going to contact online medical control (OLMC) for advice on a possible snakebite.

Although "junior" to Jon in professional rank and formal education, Rhonda had years of experience and was well respected in the ambulance service. When she heard Jon was preparing to contact OLMC, she turned to him and said, "You aren't actually considering transporting this stinking, crap-covered drunk in our ambulance, are you?"

Intimidated but not deterred, Jon told Rhonda that he simply wanted to confirm what the signs of a snakebite were with the nurse at OLMC, and he made the radio call, which took place on a recorded channel. Critical Care Nurse Gill Hoake took the call from Jon. When Jon gave the age and condition

(continues)

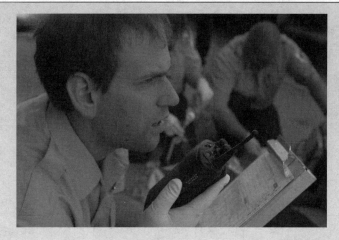

of the patient, as well as their location, Nurse Hoake reported later that he immediately knew the patient was William Bidzil. A partial transcript of the call follows:

Morton: " ... his vitals are normal with a slightly elevated heart rate, he is sweating profusely [the outside temperature at 11:30 PM was still 87° F], and he has deep scratches to both arms from the wrists to his elbows. In addition, he says he was bitten by a snake."

Hoake: "Do you see any evidence of a snakebite?"

Morton: "No, well, I've never had a snakebite. He has these deep scratches."

Hoake: "You'd know a snakebite if you saw one. Do you see any puncture wounds?"

Morton: "No punctures, but deep scratches. ... I'm not certain here."

Hoake: "Well, if you don't see any punctures, he probably wasn't bitten by a snake."

Morton: "But this isn't his normal response when he's intoxicated. We are familiar with this patient, and this ... this isn't his normal condition. He has defecated on himself and lost bladder control, and he is shaking."

Hoake: "It sounds like intoxication to me. Are you going to take him to detox?"

Morton: "My hands are full here. ... I'll call you back if we need you."

Hoake: "Copy that, have a good night."

At this point, with his experienced EMT partner and the nurse at OLMC both doubting there was a bite injury, Jon elected to load the patient into the plastic rear seat of a patrol car for the trip down to the detoxification center.

At 3:07 AM, Paramedic Jon Morton and his partner were called to the detox center on a reported cardiac arrest. Upon arrival, they saw staff members doing cardiopulmonary resuscitation (CPR) on William Bidzil. The crew attempted resuscitation, and then transported Bidzil to the local hospital, where he was pronounced dead. The cause was attributed to a fatal rattlesnake bite of the *Crotalus* species.

> As Jon and Rhonda prepared to go off shift at 8 AM, they were notified to report to the local police station for questioning, where Jon was grilled about his actions the previous evening. As he walked out of the police station, he was met by his supervisor, who placed him on paid administrative leave pending the outcome of an internal investigation.
>
> Over the next few days, local media reports harshly criticized the ambulance service and the actions of Paramedic Morton. An editorial in the local paper called for someone to be "held accountable" for Bidzil's death. Five days after the incident, the owner of the ambulance company held a press conference at which he announced that EMT Miotta was punished by being placed on a 30-day unpaid leave and Paramedic Jon Morton was fired. "We want to make sure this never happens again," the owner was quoted as saying.

A Stronger Foundation for CRM: Establishing a Just Culture

As was mentioned earlier, implementing an open communication model such as crew resource management (CRM) first requires that a solid organizational culture be built. Chapter 2 discussed how organizational stories are created and how they can negatively affect communication by causing embarrassment, intimidation, or hindsight bias that prevent individuals from speaking out, even in emergency situations.

The next foundational piece for building a resilient, open communication culture is introducing and embracing new methods of understanding human error. Placing individual blame might satisfy those seeking "someone to hold accountable," but it often only serves to hide the real source of the error and drives errors and mistakes underground. No individual within an organization that places blame will self-report a mistake for fear of the repercussions. The creation of an intentional, just, learning culture promotes open communication and cultivates higher reliability within teams, allowing CRM to be used most effectively.

Placing Blame

Placing blame for error is an understandable reaction to any untoward event. Social norms in U.S. culture are strongly biased toward holding someone responsible when something goes wrong. Unfortunately, a disturbing trend of criminalizing human errors that are made during complex events exists. After all the facts are known, it is easy to see whether a **decision point**, an action selected during the critical event, was the deciding factor that led to the crash, death, or injury. Organizations (and the public) somehow believe that everything should be under the control of the operator, regardless of the situation he or she faces.

Jobs associated with suppressing fires, catching criminals, performing high-risk surgery, and caring for the critically ill are significantly different from jobs building bridges and designing high-rise buildings. The expectations that the work will be error free are the same, however. If a building collapses or a bridge falls down, someone, somewhere is at fault; there obviously was a design flaw. If a patient suddenly and unexpectedly dies, or a building burns down when it seemed like such a small fire, or a robber is shot when he is unarmed, the public assumes that someone must be at fault. Somewhere there was a failure of risk management, and if that's so, there must be a person to blame. But can these different types of work be evaluated in the same way? Can individuals or teams be expected to perform flawlessly within dynamic, changing environments that are often personally dangerous and complex? In other words, should police work be viewed the same as bridge building? (See **FIGURE 3.1**.)

The answer is no. Individuals and teams that work in highly dynamic environments that include elements of danger and uncertainty are commonly forced to make decisions when they have only part of the available information. Clarity in their actions comes only retrospectively, after the outcome is known.

In such situations, then, what is an acceptable rate of error? When errors are made, what are individual and organizational responsibilities for making things right? How could the case of Paramedic Morton have been handled differently?

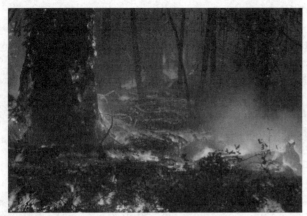

FIGURE 3.1 Danger and uncertainty often force decisions in dynamic situations.

What Is a Just Culture?

People who find themselves in the midst of an investigation of a bad outcome usually only want the truth to come out. And the truth, in their mind, is the entire story associated with the event, including the decisions they had to make, the environment they were in when the decisions were made, the organizational culture in which they were operating, the tools at hand, their education and its limits, their knowledge of the situation, their experience, and multiple other factors that are at play every time they face a similar set of circumstances. Finding the whole truth, however, is not always what a traditional investigation is about.

In the snakebite case involving Paramedic Morton, the owner of the ambulance company sincerely thought he was solving the problem by firing the person in charge, Paramedic Morton. No attention was paid to the different levels of experience each medic had, and neither was Nurse Hoake's influence taken into consideration. Additionally, during a retrospective review conducted by an outside company hired by Paramedic Morton's lawyers, investigators found that no company training related to snakebites had ever been offered, no protocols on how to handle snakebites existed, no previous cases of snakebite had occurred in more than 10 years (therefore, no "organizational story" on how to deal with them existed), and no equipment was on board the ambulance to deal with snakebites.

Neither the hospital nor the OLMC nurse were scrutinized, which is surprising considering the transcript of the call placed by Paramedic Morton. Paramedic Morton had seen this patient 27 times in the past few months. Morton told Nurse Hoake that this "wasn't [Bidzil's] normal response when he's intoxicated. ... " If anyone would know the patient's normal response when intoxicated, it would be the paramedic who saw him more than two dozen times in three months.

Yes, everyone makes mistakes. But how do organizations maintain the public trust, take responsibility for errors, sustain an open reporting and communication environment, and yet still protect themselves and their employees from being sued or professionally ruined? This is a tall order. If they work to develop a culture that allows error, continually analyzes organizational behavior and its effect on others, regularly performs in-depth critiques after both good and bad outcomes, and takes responsibility for mistakes without demeaning the individual or team that made the error they have started the process that leads to a resilient and open just culture.

There are many different perspectives on exactly what constitutes a **just culture**. Team leaders can start creating a just culture by exchanging anger at the outcome for fairness and explanation. They should take a holistic, systematic approach to trying to understand precisely why an individual or a team made the decision or series of decisions that led to what is viewed retrospectively as an undesired outcome.

Additionally, leaders must hold individuals in the organization accountable for purposeful, intentionally bad behavior. If they overlook or ignore those who intentionally try to sabotage relationships or reputations, and those who disregard well-constructed and relevant policies and procedures, their employees who strive to follow the rules, continually learn, and play fair will eventually become resentful. These employees might think, "Why should I work to build functional relationships when those who behave badly are allowed to poison the organizational well?" It has been said that reputations are built on many actions and lost through only one. Individuals find it exceedingly difficult to maintain a positive outlook and culture when one or two people behave in a manner that "undoes" all the positive contributions of many.

A just culture, so important to building the internal organizational atmosphere that allows for open communication, includes both forgiveness and understanding in the face of error (even egregious ones) and corrective action and **accountability** for those who purposefully behave in a way that is incongruent with the beliefs of the organization and its customers. Accountability describes the act of taking responsibility, being answerable and blameworthy for actions taken with the expectation of being called to account.

What Is Accountability?

Accountability is vitally important. The public has a vested interest in the performance of its emergency providers, and they need to know whether organizations understand the consequences of their mistakes. More important, they want to know whether responders learn from mistakes. Calls for accountability are really about trust. The expectations of the public are not met if a person or organization hides the facts, delays reporting, or otherwise behaves in a manner that arouses suspicion. Accountability, however, need not look like blame. If the incident analysis is done properly, when an organization takes responsibility for its actions, the bonds between the public and the organization can be strengthened and trust increased.

Accountability is directly related to the organizational and individual steps taken to learn from a mistake. Questions must be answered, information should be carefully gathered, outside expertise should be sought, impartial members of the public should be brought into the process, and those affected should know at the outset that the organization is doing everything it can to learn from the situation. Rarely do people act intentionally to create a situation in which someone is hurt or killed or property is damaged. For an organization to be accountable to the public, then, it must answer the question, "Why did the 'normal' functioning of the system create such a bad outcome?"

In the case of William Bidzil, Paramedic Morton was acting within a normally functioning system. It was not a system he created, and with only three months on the job, he arguably had made few contributions to the organizational culture that he inherited. The termination of Paramedic Morton was quick and easy, and it took the heat off the organization. But was it really a move toward accountability?

In the Bidzil case, for the ambulance company to be accountable to the public it would have analyzed a multitude of system issues that all contributed to the outcome. It would have made an open report to the public that included recommendations on how frequent system abusers should be managed, proposals for additional training related to venomous creatures of the local desert, additions of appropriate equipment and relevant protocols, and suggestions to improve many other factors related to human performance in similar situations. It's unlikely that any investigation seeking the truth behind what happened would have recommended termination of Paramedic Morton because he did not act maliciously or with purposeful intent to harm his patient.

Complacency Kills

On Friday night, January 6, 2006, prominent *New York Times* reporter David Rosenbaum was mugged and struck in the head while walking in Washington, D.C. With Rosenbaum unconscious on the sidewalk, an emergency medical services (EMS) response was initiated when someone called 9-1-1. What happened next illustrates the dangers of complacency: An engine company staffed with a crew of fire fighter/EMTs responded to the scene, and after assessing Rosenbaum, they assumed he was intoxicated. As a result of multiple miscues and delays, it took more than an hour to get Rosenbaum to the hospital, and because of poor communication between EMS and hospital staff, it was seven hours more before he underwent surgery to relieve the bleeding in his brain. He did not survive surgery.

David Rosenbaum was killed by complacency—by the "normal operations" of a system in need of repair. Complacency occurs when the organization's mission becomes unclear or is not reinforced and a condition called **normalization of deviance** develops. Normalization of deviance is a long-term phenomenon in which individuals or teams repeatedly accept a lower standard of performance until that lower standard becomes the norm. Usually this occurs because a team is operating under budget constraints or with performance standards that make deviating from protocol, policy, or process favorable. Examples of constraints include system stressors such as a high call volume or a limited number of ambulances.

Often the team or individual perceives that it would be too difficult to adhere to the higher standard when the stresses of the system are present. So, the underperforming behavior becomes the norm even after the stress passes or more resources are available. Normalization of deviance is not an individual problem, and neither is it a behavioral attribute that causes people to take actions that are purposefully harmful. The fire fighter/EMTs who responded in the Rosenbaum case were not the root cause of the incident. If the crew was held as incompetent and cited as the single defining cause of this terrible outcome, the system would have continued on in its current state, awaiting the next victim. (See **FIGURE 3.2**.)

In fire and emergency services, much like in medicine, responders are taught to assume they are dealing with the worst-case scenario and to work backward to avoid missing any life-threatening or unstable conditions that can result in a catastrophic loss. Why was this protocol not followed for Rosenbaum? One of the first steps in resolving normalization of deviance is to develop a more comprehensive outlook of the situation, one that takes a systematic and fair approach and fosters open communication.

Deviations from Protocol

To determine the root causes of complacency, team leaders must discover the systemic issues that factor in decision making. To determine systemic causes of human behavior, it is important to ask why, as in "Why would the individual or team act in a way that led to the undesired outcome?" Typically, leaders must ask

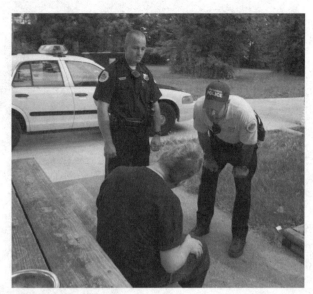

FIGURE 3.2 Complacency may be a symptom of a system in need of repair.

why continually until they are satisfied that they have uncovered as many causal factors as possible. Once leaders understand systemic causes, they can start crafting interventions designed to minimize the chances that personnel will make the same mistake in the future. (Notice that leaders should *minimize* the chances, not *eliminate*. It isn't possible to eliminate all factors that cause errors in dynamic environments; teams can only hope to work continually toward improvement.)

In the Rosenbaum case, the patient's closed head injury was downplayed by the EMTs, and they mistook him for an intoxicated patient. The crew's failure to evaluate blood pressure and assess for a closed head injury meant they were not thinking of the situation from the worst-case-scenario perspective. The crew's assumption that Rosenbaum was "passed out drunk" then led them to perform a series of other actions that critically delayed proper care for Rosenbaum. In retrospect, these decisions and actions were deviations from protocol and accepted standards of care. It might be assumed that the crew intentionally deviated from protocol, knowing the outcome could be fatal, but that assumption would likely be wrong and might also prevent the organization from performing a deeper analysis.

The crew that responded to the 9-1-1 call for Rosenbaum typically encountered several intoxicated patients each shift, and the demand for ambulances in their busy EMS system influenced their decision process. The crew's decision to interpret the situation as a low severity incident may have been a complacent response. Again, this is not intentional behavior; it's automatic and practiced. To fight complacency team leaders can call attention to the biases personnel develop regarding frequently seen patients and remind personnel through the use of stories (outcomes that are rich in detail) what can happen if they become complacent. This type of organizational intervention, when mixed with an open communication model such as CRM, can work very well to reduce complacency.

For example, for a number of reasons, it is not uncommon for EMS personnel to become complacent and to miss important cues related to a patient's condition. However, if an individual is part of a team that uses an effective communication model such as CRM, some protection against complacency is offered. CRM relies on all team members to provide input, inquire, and challenge each other. In a healthy CRM environment, complacency is uncommon.

One decision the engine crew made was to determine that the patient was not critically injured. Another was to order a nonemergency transport ambulance. This second decision, of course, was based on the first assumption. How could this occur? Leaders must again ask why: Why order a nonemergency ambulance? Perhaps an organizational story led them to this decision.

As mentioned earlier, the Washington, D.C., EMS system is extremely busy, and ambulances are in high demand. Perhaps in a previous case the EMT-Basic crew members ordered Advanced Life Support Paramedic ambulances to respond on an emergent basis to an unconscious patient. The unconscious patient, however, turned out to be intoxicated. What story is created from such an incident? Someone redirected critical resources to the side of a drunk. This story becomes a cultural barrier against taking emergent action for suspected drunks, and it also helps reinforce the bias that Rosenbaum's situation was not an emergency.

When younger team members are influenced to deviate from protocol or standards by veteran crew members it is termed **veteran's bias**. Veterans' decisions, as discussed in the last chapter, often are driven by positive or negative organizational stories. Veteran's bias commonly occurs in front-loaded EMS systems that use engine companies as first responders to screen patients for transport. The culture can become such that the patients must prove to the crew that they are sick and require an ambulance. This, again, is a system problem, not one that can be corrected by punishing the field operators.

Establishing and Losing Trust

After the Rosenbaum incident was analyzed from many sides and by multiple parties, the various causal factors became fairly well understood. In this particular case, a lawsuit led to a comprehensive settlement agreement and a host of system changes that were necessary. When organizations harm someone, they owe that person or his or her representatives a settlement—not to make them whole, but to acknowledge the loss and help with future hardship. More important than money, they owe the person the truth, an apology, a comprehensive analysis of the system that caused the failure, and a promise to implement substantive actions to improve the system. Only this type of response allows organizations to build trust with the public, and only through trust can teams focus on the failures of the system and not the individual.

In the Rosenbaum case, however, trust was not easily gained. The initial comments made by senior authorities gave the public reason to question whether the agency really wanted to understand what happened, or whether it was more interested in making excuses and covering up mistakes. At first, the public was told "at no time did he [Rosenbaum] present symptoms or detectable injuries that would cause first responders to request the addition of advanced life support resources." But, according to the facts of the case, on arrival the crew assessed Rosenbaum and assigned him a Glasgow Coma Scale (GCS) rating of 6. This rating system ranges from GCS-3, which identifies the patient as completely comatose, to GCS-15, which identifies the patient as awake and fully oriented. In most systems, a rating of lower than GCS-8 is an indication to provide advanced airway treatment and place a breathing tube down the patient's trachea.

The initial report concluded, "Our operational review indicates that appropriate measures were taken and EMS providers met all standards of care as outlined in our protocols."[1] That may have indeed been the case. However, if the crew met all standards of care as outlined in the protocols, and the death was preventable, then mustn't there be a system problem? Public trust could have been established in this case if the agency had issued a response that accepted responsibility for the undesired outcome and promised to make an all-out effort to understand the human errors involved. The agency did not do this.

These types of cases are the crucible in which a just culture is validated and culturally accepted within an agency. Unfortunately, for many organizations they are opportunities lost.

CASE STUDY 2

The Rock Creek Tavern was a very popular place. Built in the 1930s, the lodge-style building in the hills outside Portland, Oregon, commonly drew large crowds on the weekends. By the time the fire was reported, flames were consuming the entire back portion of the building and threatening nearby structures. Fire companies that arrived called for a total of three alarms, and more than 60 fire fighters fought the blaze at one point. Unfortunately, the building was a total loss. The fire, however, was only the beginning of a story that would challenge the just culture of the large fire department responsible for fighting it.

As the fire equipment returned to their stations during the early morning hours, another emergency call was received just a few miles down the road from the ravaged tavern. A vehicle had left the road and struck a utility pole, and the driver was critically injured. Some of the same fire units that responded to the fire rolled to the accident, where paramedics quickly removed the victim for transport to a trauma center. As the fire fighters extricated the victim, they noticed that a 100-ft (30.5-m) roll of 5-in.-diameter (127-mm-diameter) fire hose weighing more than 100 lbs (45.4 kg) was partially jammed under the damaged vehicle.

It was evident that the hose, belonging to one of the fire engines that had recently left the fire scene, had fallen off the rear of the fire engine into the street. To those present, the cause of the accident was clear: The driver had lost control of his car after the car struck the heavy fire hose in the

(continues)

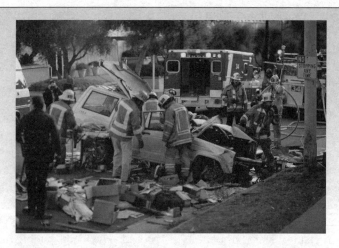

road. The patient's condition deteriorated, and he died before he arrived at the trauma center.

The Right Reaction: Taking Responsibility

What type of individual and organizational response is appropriate in a just culture after such an incident as presented in Case Study 2? Admitting an error should be a nonpunitive event within such a system. For a just culture to work, personnel must know that revealing an error is paramount to the learning process and future safety of the organization and other personnel. They must feel safe revealing details and honestly providing an accounting of what happened, without fear of reprisal. Admitting error and taking responsibility defuse the event and move the group, community, and organization past the event. (See **FIGURE 3.3**.)

For this fire department, the response was immediate. The fire chief and his executive staff met in the early morning hours, put together incident management and accident analysis teams, and prepared a press release. By the time the morning news was broadcast and commuters were sipping their coffee on the way to work, the word was out. The basics of the press release were as follows: A tragic accident occurred following the fire. A person died. It appears the person struck one of our fire hoses, and it appears to be our fault. We are allowing a third-party to complete a crash reconstruction, and we are also conducting an immediate internal analysis to see what went wrong so that we can learn from this terrible event.

A just culture is about determining a cause for failure that satisfies both the demand for accountability and the need for learning and improvement. This act by the fire department was a large step in gaining public trust. Openly taking responsibility organizationally and immediately relieves the pressure of trying to hide investigative actions behind a curtain of suspicion. Modeling appropriate behavior is key. In doing so, the organization writes a story, one that says the right thing to do is to be honest and to communicate openly to gain trust. Effective CRM requires open, honest, and respectful communication. For CRM to take hold in an organization, the organizational environment must be such that individuals feel a responsibility to do the right thing, to speak up when they see a problem, and to commit themselves to continual improvement.

Postincident Analysis

When a comprehensive postincident analysis is performed in a just culture, the individuals conducting the analysis understand that no single account is the one true story of what happened. From this perspective, the investigators come to understand the event better and can identify multiple causal factors. Then, plans can

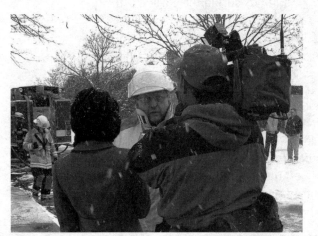

FIGURE 3.3 Only by telling the truth can an organization gain the public's trust.

be made to provide the necessary education, systems changes, or equipment purchases that will minimize the chances of repeating the same mistakes.

Systemic Cause Analysis

To establish a culture that embraces error as part of learning, team leaders must understand the fundamentals associated with fair and comprehensive incident analysis. Using a systemic approach to analyzing incidents and accidents means that teams must evaluate all individual and team actions in the context of the entirety—the culture, the specific situation, personnel training, and experience levels—everything. When investigating and creating causal diagrams, individual actions and decisions should not be separated from the whole to avoid distorting the actual environment that people were working in when the incident occurred. A systemic approach should perceive the accident as part of the normal operational process, not as an individual or team failure.

For the fire department involved in the hose incident, a just culture meant reviewing the incident as they did all failures by conducting a systemic cause analysis. A systemic cause analysis typically begins with asking each person involved to write down his or her perceptions of the incident. Individuals should isolate themselves and conduct a first-pass written summary free of the influence of others. What did they see and hear? Why did they do what they did? It can be helpful to ask the individuals involved simply to write a narrative of the situation, and then separate decisions and influences into the following categories:

- System influences: Influences generally associated with written and adopted policies, procedures, and rules. System influences also include organizational culture issues and the hierarchical structure. Examples include out-of-date policies, irrelevant rules, instructions that are too dense, procedures that are not memorialized in writing, and protocols that are too complicated to follow. Other examples may be cultural issues that are related to organizational stories (e.g., "this is how we do it here") and overdeference to rank.
- Education and training failures: Initial operator education was inadequate or not completely relevant, the training was not up-to-date, the training was not provided in an appropriate style for the complexity of the subject (e.g., video instead of hands on), or training was delivered using a method that did not resonate with the student (visual vs. auditory or touch).
- Circumstances beyond the operator's control: Examples include equipment breakage, weather, or bystander interference.
- Human factor influences: Examples include cognitive errors in processing information, fatigue, equipment design issues, or expert–novice influence.

Team leaders may provide a list as an example. In general, it is helpful to categorize influences to address them and assist in determining how a leader will manage the issue and who within the organization (or outside of it) will take responsibility for implementing recommendations for improvement.

There will be inconsistencies in people's stories. In the heat of battle, no one individual perceives the same information flow. Each person assigns a different level of importance to certain cues, and therefore, each may have completely different perceptions of the same incident. This is one critical reason to separate the team members when they write their original account; it helps to identify many more contributory factors than leaders would otherwise get from a collective viewpoint.

Once the appropriate reports, pictures, policies, training records, best practices documents, and interview notes have been gathered, the next step is to build an incident timeline. With the timeline, leaders can conclude when specific decisions were made by the crew.

The Basic Rules of Systemic Cause Analysis

Systemic cause analysis teams can follow a few basic guidelines to ensure success. First, it is important to make sure the right people are on the analysis team. For example, if it includes supervisory representation, then it should also have representatives from labor groups. In addition, it is important to make sure the appropriate technical experts are either present or readily on call. It is critical to include several operators, those on the front line who are on scene conducting the high-risk operations. It also helps to have someone present who knows the organizational policies.

Second, as mentioned earlier, all the relevant facts associated with the incident should be gathered. The people who were involved should be asked to write down their stories, perceptions, and actions. Experts from outside the organization should be invited, if possible, to assist in conducting the first few systemic analyses so that team leaders have an idea of how an analysis should work.

Third, team leaders should always develop, introduce, and follow basic ground rules. For example, they should state that there will be no personal attacks or introduce the concept of cognitive dissonance so that team members understand the types of intellectual and emotional factors and stress that can influence their behavior (and the behavior of others).

Finally, the organization must commit procedures to writing that everyone can understand. The organization's risk manager or safety officer, with specific direction from the fire chief, should complete this task. In addition, once the procedure is in writing, then it should be introduced to the policymakers of the organization so that they understand what is occurring when an accident happens and why it takes time to get it right.

Making the process as transparent as possible helps to build credibility and also provides critical support to the organizational leaders and policymakers in the face of media attention. Well-developed processes that describe an objective analysis of all relevant incident factors demonstrate that the organization is willing to look at everything, and everyone, involved in the incident being examined.

An Important Piece: Self-Reporting and Trend Files

Once an organization has developed a process for analyzing errors and accidents in a systematic fashion, it is helpful to create a method for individuals to self-report their errors and **near misses**. Although the term *near miss* has become part of the lexicon for aviation, EMS, and the fire service, it is somewhat misleading. What a near miss actually describes is a "near hit," something that almost caused a serious accident or injury but didn't.

Best practices for developing self-reporting systems include the following:
- Forms can be anonymously completed and submitted.
- Forms use a standardized set of questions that collect key information such as age of the operator, years of experience in current position, type of incident, and so forth.
- Forms create a foundational database so that key information can be grouped into "trend files" and used by the agency's performance improvement and risk manager teams.
- Forms are developed in a manner so that the data can be entered into larger, national databases for further study (for example, www.firefighterclosecalls.com).

As mentioned, information in near-miss databases should be collected into **trend files**, which are essentially lists that include potential accident causes, training issues, equipment issues, and other factors that can be mined from the database. For example, an EMS trend file might focus on medication errors. An organization could establish one trend file for medication errors in general, and subfiles for errors involving specific medications.

Risk managers and performance management teams may elect to set specific performance thresholds for certain types of errors. They might decide that a 90 percent success rate is acceptable for intubation to be studied and they might decide to examine every single incident involving a fire fighter injury. The severity of the incident will dictate when an investigation is in order.

Near-miss databases and trend files contribute to the learning organization, empower every employee to be a risk manager and seek out potential failure points, and reinforce the concept of nonpunitive systematic error analysis. By creating this type of system, front-line operators know that the information they contribute will help others avoid the same mistakes, and it demonstrates the open communication expected within a just culture.

A Summary of a System Failure

In the case of the fire hose incident presented in Case Study 2, the final determination was that the primary causal factors were all system influences. That fire department had a long-standing practice of carrying damaged hose back to the fire station on the rear step of the fire engine. This practice started back when fire engines had broad rear steps because the firefighters rode on the rear tailboard on their way to the fire. Whereas the rear steps had changed dramatically in size over the years, the long-standing practice of carrying rolled hose on the tailboard had not. With no policy against carrying loose equipment, no tie-downs provided by the organization, and—even more influential—a long history of no problems doing it that way, the situation was ripe for a tragedy.

The resolution was satisfactory to the public: Organizational learning occurred and the fire department took responsibility for the mistake. One part of the investigation's conclusion, however, was a surprise to fire department employees as well as the lawyers preparing to file suit against the fire department: The fire department would not make an in-depth inquiry into which individual fire engine was involved, and neither would it dig deep enough to find out who was driving the particular engine. The fire department stated that there was no reason to do so, and even under pressure from the plaintiff's attorneys, the fire department never determined who the individual driver was because to identify the person would have caused unnecessary personal anguish over what was essentially an organizational mistake.

Why Develop a Learning Culture?

Immense political pressure is placed on the leaders of most public organizations when something goes wrong. People want answers, and they want them quickly. In addition, the media is famous for jumping to half-baked conclusions and placing blame. They, after all, have to get the story out now, before the next big thing comes along and erases this event from public consciousness. When an accident or serious incident occurs, the behavior of many public agencies can be reprehensible. They will confuse the facts, defend their practices, obscure the investigative process, delay the outcomes, and simply fail to admit errors for fear of litigation (which will occur anyway), which leads the media to believe that if they don't get the story out and determine who is at fault, no one will.

Agencies that want to develop a learning culture take a different approach, one of openness, clarity, and honesty, as described earlier in this chapter. They educate their policymakers about the value of conducting systemic cause analysis, fostering a just culture, and facilitating nonpunitive self-reporting of error. They need to do this not just once, but consistently, and they can provide actual case examples of how embedding best practices in high-risk organizations works. When organizational policymakers are educated about CRM, less pressure is put on the organizational leader, and thus less pressure on the employees, when something goes wrong. Operators are allowed to perform at their best, report those things that can (or did) cause accidents and errors without fear of retribution, and learn from their mistakes.

In such an environment, the public receives honest and straightforward feedback from organizational leaders and policymakers: "We are deeply sorry. We made a serious mistake. We are examining all factors surrounding this incident so that we can understand why it happened and minimize the chance of recurrence. In the meantime, we are providing as much support to the family as possible, and we are also supporting our employees, who are understandably devastated."

In this type of culture, the organization can introduce the principles of CRM with ease. Open communication, direct and honest feedback, and collective problem solving—the hallmarks of CRM—are already part of the organizational fabric. The actual implementation of CRM and learning about individual decision-making processes becomes much easier. In constructing the cultural foundation that allows for a systemic cause analysis of errors and open feedback, team leaders should keep in mind the following points:

- A single account is never enough and cannot do justice to the complexity of events. This is particularly important to remember when analyzing team performance.
- A just culture is about compromise. As discussed earlier in Chapter 2 on organizational stories, it is vitally important to recognize the balance between rigid rules and policies and the wider context of the dynamic work environment. How the operators perceive what occurred is given the same weight as—or more than—the perceptions of those in managerial or supervisory roles.
- A just culture pays attention to the view from below. In studies of high-reliability organizations, emphasis is placed on paying attention to the views of the operator, who performs at the "sharp end," on the street and in the trenches. Operators who perform tasks on a regular basis in critical environments have a unique perspective on how they must often work around equipment, policies, or procedures that were developed for one process but that have been, over time, adapted to others.
- A just culture never uses other people to deflect blame, attention, or responsibility. Instead, it recognizes how the individual's performance, and his or her recovery from error, is critical to the team's and the organization's goals. Leaders who fail to take responsibility never achieve a just culture. Full disclosure from peers and subordinates requires trust, and people do not trust those who deflect responsibility for their own failures.
- Disclosure is paramount. Not disclosing can appear as dishonesty. Operators and practitioners are responsible for disclosing their errors, and the organization and its leaders are responsible for providing legal and professional protection for those who disclose in an honest and forthright manner. People don't fail to report because they are dishonest; they fail to report because they fear the repercussions (or the organizational story that will develop).
- Protecting disclosure and balancing it with necessary reporting (for example, for compliance purposes) is difficult. Policies must be in place that demonstrate the organization's commitment to protecting its employees and defending individuals if reported points are used out of context.

- Proportionality and decency are crucial. So is accountability for purposeful violations. In a just culture, people must see that those who openly break the rules or act maliciously are dealt with appropriately and corrective action is taken (including termination, if necessary).

Summary

In the absence of a learning culture, individuals who work in dangerous or dynamic work environments fear what will happen when they make a mistake and how they will be judged. Will anyone understand their decision process? Will they be held personally responsible for making a mistake in a dynamic situation?

Establishing a just culture and implementing a process for systemic cause analysis of accidents, errors, and mistakes enable individuals to perform without fear of retribution for honest mistakes. Employees become the most powerful tool an organization has when implementing an open communication model such as CRM. They model appropriate behavior, honestly critique their own performance, and continually suggest methods for improving operations. This is the type of behavior that, demonstrated consistently, leads to success.

Once a team leader understands the cultural foundations of organizational story, just culture, and systemic cause analysis for learning, he or she is ready to examine the decision-making process in pressure situations.

Wrap Up

Ready for Review

- Individuals and teams that work in highly dynamic environments, where there are elements of danger and uncertainty, are commonly forced to make decisions when they have only part of the available information. Clarity in their actions only comes retrospectively, after the outcome is known.
- Accountability is directly related to the organizational and individual steps that are taken to learn from a mistake.
- For a just culture to work, employees must know that revealing an error is paramount to the learning process and future safety of the organization and other personnel.
- To become embedded in organizational culture, CRM requires an environment where individuals feel a responsibility to do the right thing, to speak up when they see a problem, and to commit themselves to continual improvement.
- When a comprehensive postincident analysis is performed within the framework of a just culture, the investigators understand that no single account is the "one true" story of what happened.
- A systematic approach to error evaluation should perceive an accident as part of the "normal" operating process, not as an individual or team failure.
- Agencies with a learning culture address incidents with an air of openness, clarity, and honesty.

Vital Vocabulary

Accountability The act of taking responsibility, being answerable and blameworthy for actions taken with the expectation of being called to account.

Decision point A specific time during an event when an action is selected that influences the outcome of the event.

Just culture A culture in which a holistic, systematic approach is taken to understand precisely why an individual or team made the decision or series of decisions that led to what is viewed retrospectively as an undesired outcome.

Near miss An incident that almost caused a serious accident or injury, but didn't.

Normalization of deviance A long-term phenomenon in which individuals or teams repeatedly accept a lower standard of performance until that standard becomes the norm.

Trend files A database that contains information collected in near-miss accounts.

Veteran's bias When younger team members are influenced to deviate from established practices by veteran crew members.

Assessment in Action

1. Critical elements of a just culture include all but which one of the following?
   A. Honesty
   B. Trust
   C. Open communication
   D. Autocratic management
2. Systemic cause analysis involves which of the following items?
   A. Trend files
   B. Sentinel indicators
   C. Retrospective analysis
   D. All of the above.
3. A learning organization strives to accomplish which of the following tasks?
   A. Admitting errors
   B. Punishing mistakes as a central theme
   C. Encouraging personnel to report on other members' actions
   D. Managing errors from the top down
4. Traditional postincident error analysis focuses on
   A. forgiveness.
   B. learning from mistakes.
   C. placing blame.
   D. systemic cause analysis.

In-Classroom Activity

Allow students to discuss their perspectives of the organizational culture they are involved in. Compare and contrast the organizational culture with a just culture and a learning organization.

References

1. Colbert King, "The Death of David Rosenbaum," *The Washington Post*, February 25, 2006.

4

The Critical Decision Process

Objectives

- Describe the role of conflict in the decision-making process.
- Describe the role of CRM in an event-driven scenario.
- Describe the risks and rewards of the decision-making process.

CASE STUDY 1

Gunther Foss, age 54, climbed the 85-foot-tall (25.9-meter-tall) Douglas fir tree in his backyard intending to trim off the top 20 ft (6.1 m) or so, which had been damaged in a recent windstorm. He carried with him an electric chainsaw with a 14-in. (35.6-cm) blade, which was connected to his house by a 100-foot-long (30.5-meter-long) extension cord he had plugged into an exterior outlet on his deck. As Gunther completed his cut, the top of the tree fell away from his house and toward a set of Bonneville Power feeder lines that ran through an easement behind his house. When the top of the tree struck the uppermost line, more than 100,000 volts coursed through the tree, through Gunther, and down the cord into his house.

Gunther's wife Kara, inside working in the kitchen, first thought a car had slammed into their residence. The sudden explosion of electricity caused flames to shoot from every electrical outlet in the house. Kara ran out the front door as the electrical panel exploded, immediately setting the house on fire. While Gunther slumped gravely injured 60 ft (18.3 m) up the tree in the backyard, unable to yell for help, his wife called 9-1-1 and reported that their house had "just exploded" and was "on fire."

Arriving fire fighters quickly extinguished the flames and subsequently found the burned electrical cord leading into the tall tree in the backyard. As fire fighters followed the cord over to the tree, they looked up and saw Gunther draped over a branch. More alarmingly, the fire fighters discovered that the top of the tree was still in contact with the high-voltage lines. Gunther desperately needed to be rescued before he fell or before another charge came through the lines. Kara, now discovering along with the fire fighters that her husband was gravely injured and 60 ft up in the tree, immediately started pleading with the rescuers to "get Gunther down from there." Neighbors gathered along the fence line in the backyard, offering advice and yelling suggestions.

Lieutenant Warren Parks and his crew from Ladder 56 were met by Battalion Chief Dan Aspen in the backyard. Within minutes, they were joined by Officer Peak from the local police department, who was asked to assist Kara back into the front yard where she wouldn't be in danger from the rescue operation or any discharges from the nearby power lines. As she was led away, Chief Aspen, Lieutenant Parks, and the members of Ladder 56 engaged in a robust discussion regarding how to best stabilize the situation until the power company could arrive and cut the electricity in the lines.

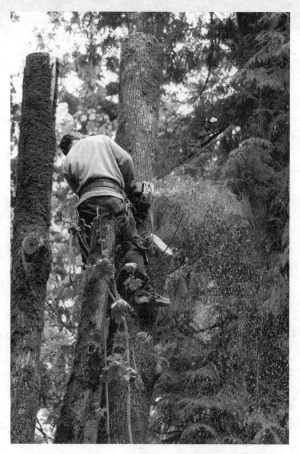

Understanding a Complex Process

The intention of this chapter is to describe some of the many factors that can influence the way teams make decisions while working in dynamic environments. For example, **conflict** has a powerful and important role, particularly because it produces an emotional response that can sharpen the senses and help team members and leaders develop a curiosity about alternative views. Conflict describes an actual or perceived opposition of needs, values, and interests. Of course, if not properly managed, conflict can also sabotage the best efforts of any team.

Additionally, the experience of team members and the urgency of the situation profoundly affect the way a team makes decisions. Decision making is different for novices than it is for veterans. The process is slower and more rule-oriented for novices, whereas for the veteran intuition plays a much larger role. In urgent situations, teams tend to trade accuracy and safety for speed and efficiency. Only after the incident is over do they have the luxury of recognizing whether the trade-off was worthwhile.

The Role of Conflict

In Gunther's backyard, the team dynamics were intense. Each person, whether they were a fire fighter, police officer, or chief, had different experiences with electrical emergencies. In addition, no clear policies were available to instruct on which actions were appropriate, the power company had reported that it had an estimated time of arrival of more than 30 minutes, and neighbors and family continually voiced their opinions that the fire crews should immediately rescue Gunther before he fell and died.

Essentially, this was a classic situation where time pressure and circumstances beyond the control of the operators could affect the quality of the decision process.

As options and alternatives were discussed, it became apparent that polarized viewpoints were in play. Some fire fighters and command staff were visibly upset that alternatives to waiting were even being discussed at all; talking about options, in their view, breached any safe practice they could conceive. Although the crews on scene knew that the power in the large feeder lines was temporarily interrupted, no one knew for how long. Others believed that not discussing the alternatives would force crews into accepting a single course of action, even if the situation were to change. (What if the tree branch were to become dislodged? What if he were to fall part way down and become accessible from the ground? How would fire fighters safely approach that situation, or could they? Was there a safe way to dislodge the tree branch from the power line without directly contacting it?)

Regardless of organizational culture, individual and team conflicts are evident to the untrained eye simply by observing body language, facial expression, and behaviors among peers. Even the word *conflict* conjures up visions of fights, raised voices, and tense verbal exchanges. However, if conflict is well managed, it can be a very healthy attribute in teams. Conflicting viewpoints are a normal part of the decision-making process during a dynamic situation. Because it is impossible to know the actual outcome (not the desired one), it's inevitable that each individual will determine his or her own method to manage the situation effectively.

If the culture is healthy and embraces open, respectful communication, another significant behavior is recognized: ready dialogue between all team members, including those who have hierarchal standing within the group. A good team understands conflict, its role in the decision process, and its importance in vetting alternatives. The key is to keep the dialogue respectful and not personalize the differences in opinion.

Effective team members will establish a curiosity about their own behavior and about the behavior of their cohorts and their leader. Instead of simply reacting negatively to comments or suggestions, someone with a healthy curiosity asks himself or herself, "Why is this person, suggestion, or comment upsetting me? What am I holding on to or trying to defend? What is the perspective of my teammate, and why does that person see things differently?" By developing the ability to ask these questions, a team member can depersonalize the conversation. Proposals by other team members that conflict with that team member's "reality" cease to become a personal challenge and instead help him or her develop a shared understanding of the entire situation.

In some situations a team member's suggestion will not be used, and instead the team decides on a different course of action. If the tactic employed by the team is unsuccessful, it is important that the team member maintain a sense of support and not negatively comment about the undesired outcome. Teamwork is sharing both success and failure, and allowing those who err to preserve their dignity strengthens team bonds. Additionally, the other team members will be more likely to support that person when he or she inevitably make a mistake.

Conflict brings out the alternatives, emphasizes goals and objectives, and allows the team to come to a shared understanding of what needs to be done. As the event unfolds, those who are able to maintain their curiosity about their behavior and that of others will see that healthy conflicting views and respectful interaction provide the collective situational awareness needed by a high-performance team.

Event-Driven Scenarios and CRM

Emergency scenes are *event-driven* scenarios. This means that every situation unfolds in a manner that is relatively unpredictable and that the tempo of events is not entirely under the control of the operators on scene. (See **FIGURE 4.1**.) In addition, each person viewing the exact same scene will have a slightly different perspective, based in part on that person's area of expertise, level of experience, quality of training, ability to recall applicable written procedures, and personal context. Any group on an emergency scene does, however, share two significant realities: No one knows exactly how the situation will unfold, and neither do they know the outcome.

The previous two chapters discussed the cultural foundation that is necessary for establishing an open communication model such as crew resource management (CRM). Once a solid foundation has been laid, it is important for each individual front-line operator to more fully understand how people make decisions, both as individuals and when part of a high-performance team. High-performance teams work best when they have a collective understanding of the situation that they face. Effective CRM ensures that every member of the team has an appreciation of the following key points:

- The exact nature of the problem, its cause, and any confounding or complicating factors
- The skills, strengths, weaknesses, and experience of their fellow team members
- An understanding of what is likely to happen based on taking no action
- An understanding of what is likely to happen if the team chooses a specific action
- A shared knowledge of the desired outcome
- A shared strategy, with an understanding of what tactics need to be accomplished, by whom, and when

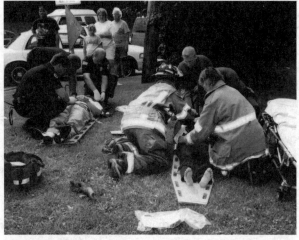

FIGURE 4.1 Event-driven scenarios unfold in unpredictable ways.

- The knowledge that any member of the team, regardless of rank or experience, can respectfully question the strategy and/or provide additional cues that will help the team gain a better understanding of the situation as it unfolds

Only when the team truly knows how to use CRM can it maximize the potential for a successful outcome. Gaining the ability to develop and cultivate a shared vision among team members is a skill that requires practice and knowledge of how the human mind works while under pressure to make a decision. Unlike in domains where operators have the benefit of time and know that an outcome will be the same every time they apply a set of rules and procedures, emergency work is extremely dynamic. Operators cannot know every factor influencing the emergency situation before they must make a decision, and they must be able to adjust and adapt as the situation unfolds. Team members should know when and how to slow the decision process to gain a better perspective.

Key Factors in Decision-Making Efforts

Decisions are often driven by one of several human performance behaviors. Each one provides a measure of **cognitive control** that can be either beneficial or unhelpful, depending on how and when it is used. Cognitive control describes the collection of brain processes that are responsible for planning, cognitive flexibility, abstract thinking, rule acquisition, initiating appropriate actions and inhibiting inappropriate actions, and selecting relevant sensory information. For understanding how the decision process affects CRM, two of the most commonly used methods for making decisions should be looked at: rule-based analysis and recognition-primed decision making.

Rule-Based Decisions

Rule-based analysis of probabilities is a labor-intensive exercise that can be very helpful when a team is faced with a problem to solve and plenty of time to solve it. The problem may be complex or simple, but the element of time allows the team to evaluate many different options and arrive at a solution that poses the smallest risk while delivering the largest benefit. Rule-based analyses are conducted to capture the knowledge of domain experts into expressions that can be evaluated and known as rules. These rules can be compiled into a rule base so that operators can evaluate current working conditions against the rule base and chain rules together until they reach a conclusion.

Most written operating protocols and rules are developed through a comprehensive knowledge-based process. Best practices are developed for a specific situation and a given set of circumstances. When committed to writing, this is often represented in a clearly defined procedure that says, "If A happens, then do B. If C happens, then do D and E. In any event, always do X and be aware of Y." This is the general format for many procedures, and it helps front-line operators develop a sense of what is important when facing a specific scenario. In many situations that can develop relatively slowly, such as a hazardous materials or mass casualty incidents (compared to a structure fire or cardiac arrest, that is), with the little bit of extra time operators have, they can quickly review checklists and procedures that can be very helpful in such low-frequency, high-risk events. However, knowledge-based solutions are only marginally helpful as dynamic operating guidelines because every situation is unique.

For example, a knowledge-based protocol for treating a diabetic can provide specific medication dosage information, and it can also help the operator recognize important cues when dealing with a diabetic. However, regardless of how well thought out the protocol, it can never anticipate all the factors that come into play on scene, in real life. The patient may be taking any one of hundreds of medications, may have several other disease processes that affect the underlying condition, or the person may be the victim of a traumatic injury. No protocol can be developed to deal with all these contingencies, and if someone attempted to do so, it would be so complex that it would be impossible to commit to memory. Therefore, the best of these procedures provide *cue recognition*, or a series of things that front-line operators must pay attention to during the event.

When teams try to solve something they haven't faced before, deal with the unfamiliar, or approach a highly complex situation, using the knowledge-based process alone can be prone to error. In a dynamically developing situation, factors over which teams have no control influence the outcome. In these cases, using a recognition-primed process allows more adaptability.

Recognition-Primed Decision Making

A **recognition-primed decision** process is quick, effective decision making by operators when they are faced with complex situations. In this model, the decision maker is assumed to generate a possible course of action, compare it to the constraints imposed by the situation, and select the first course of action that is not rejected. It is typically developed over time within a certain domain (such as firefighting or emergency nursing). Front-line operators gain personal expertise through continuous exposure to certain situations. In addition, by regularly applying the experience gained during these situations to real-life and training scenarios, they solidify their use of certain decision and motor skills. Their intuitive sense of what works and what doesn't drives them to create "rules," or ready-made solutions to problems that can be applied any time they encounter a situation that is similar to one they have previously come across. Typically, when the situation doesn't perfectly fit the rule (and it rarely is an ideal fit), the experienced front-line operator modifies the strategy as things develop.

Making decisions, regardless of threat, depends on four factors: information, experience, knowledge, and urgency. Making rapid, correct decisions on the fire ground or during a medical emergency requires operators to rapidly process the information and potential situation they face and formulate an action plan. Studies have shown that experienced operators in emergency situations make decisions using this unique adapted behavior of recognizing a situation and applying a rule that previously worked. Hence the term *recognition-primed decision making*.

Because front-line operators cannot fully analyze all options during a critical and dynamic situation, and they are under time compression to act quickly and decisively, they develop a coherent strategy based on their current understanding of the situation, regardless of whether it is complete. This technique, also known as *pattern matching*, allows them to apply a previously used rule and/or use skill and intuition to manage the current scenario.

Importantly, this is a skill that is unique to experienced veterans. Novices rely far more on the printed procedures and protocols because they have little experience to draw from. The metaphor of a hard drive has been used in the past: A novice's hard drive, essentially, contains only the basic programs available. The veteran's hard drive stores not only the basic programs, but also many stories of past successes and failures through which the veteran can readily sift during an emergent decision-making situation. This provides balance and value to a team—the varied experiences that team members have, written policies, organizational culture, the stories of success and failure (team members' and others')—all supply a rich background for high-performance teams.

Consider the case of Gunther, up in the tree. When crews arrived, the electrical power to the lines was off, disconnected by a breaker in the line that interrupted the electrical flow when the branch struck the power line. However, the emergency crews have no way of knowing how long the breaker will stay open. They don't know whether it resets automatically or is reset manually. They don't know whether Gunther will stay draped over the branch or whether the wind will pick up and toss him to the ground.

The novice knows the department has no protocol or policy specific to this particular situation. The protocol on electrical emergencies includes information related to underground vaults, electrical fires, and safe operating distances, but it doesn't mention high-voltage lines or automatic breakers. The high-angle rescue protocol doesn't consider conducting an operation within an electrically charged tree. The burn and spinal immobilization protocols reveal nothing on how to maintain spinal integrity while evacuating a severely injured person high off the ground in a tree.

The veteran knows what she did in the past. She knows that the last time she dealt with a high-power line at a wildland fire, the power company told her that the breakers could be reengaged at any time through an automatic process. She also understands pressure and is able to withstand the urgency being expressed by bystanders.

Veteran front-line operators understand that when operating within a dangerous and dynamic environment, decision making can be divided into two general categories—life threatening and non-life threatening. Decision makers can make non-life-threatening decisions when they have time to evaluate options. They can accomplish this in an unhurried manner and can choose the best option based on a risk-benefit analysis. Life-threatening decisions do not offer such leisurely reflection.

So, are the decisions regarding Gunther life threatening or not? Is there time to consider options, weigh outcomes, and develop a safety plan, or do the front-line operators need to act immediately? Veterans become veterans because they understand how to manage risk. They know how to mitigate a situation and manage the decision process while maintaining the safest possible environment for them and for their team. They learn to purposefully slow down the situation to relieve some of the time compression. Veterans recognize that there are certain situations in which time compression is forced upon them and they have to act fast to save a life, but they also recognize that teams often inappropriately act before thinking—they compress time when it isn't necessary.

Three key factors mentioned earlier can ensure that teams can implement effective CRM:

- An understanding of what is likely to happen based on taking no action
- An understanding of what is likely to happen if the team chooses a specific action
- A shared knowledge of the desired outcome

When team members understand the decision process, they are better prepared to evaluate their own gut-level tendency to take action, or to "compress time." If the team is to gain a collective awareness of the situation, they need to know the answers to the preceding questions: What can happen if the team lengthens the time for decision making and takes no action? What could occur (good and bad) if the team takes a specific action? What are the desired outcomes?

Again, consider Gunther Foss's situation, up in the tree. The team must deliberate what is likely to happen if it takes the power company 30 minutes or more to respond. The team collectively understands that Gunther is unlikely to survive if he falls or if the power comes back on and reenergizes the tree, and that he might even succumb to his serious burn injuries. However, by taking no action, the team would remain relatively safe.

The team must also consider the pressures to continue, to compress time, to "do something." Gunther's wife is screaming in the front yard and boisterous bystanders are commenting on the fire fighters' lack of bravery. It took a strong team and a determined leader to discuss options but not immediately act. This is the value of CRM. With CRM, your team gains a collective awareness of the situation, understands the risks of action, the risks of no action, and the potential outcome of your strategic decisions. Regardless of members' rank or experience, a high-performance team maximizes its value by openly communicating the "why" behind every decision.

In Gunther Foss's situation, the fire fighters determined that there were no viable options other than to wait for the power company. Their experience was enriched, however, by the open discussion that occurred and by struggling to find alternative, yet safe methods to intervene. During the postincident analysis, those who tend to think in a linear, procedurally based fashion needed to be reassured that discussing alternatives doesn't mean alternatives will be acted upon, but that discussion of potential options can empower those in the team to think differently and to be better prepared the next time they encounter such a situation. For those who process in a less linear manner, the results of the decision affirmed the importance of having people on the team who are less action-oriented and more prone to analyzing before acting. Gunther survived; his tree didn't.

Decision Process Risks and Rewards

Teams often develop patterns and rules that they can apply to dynamic environments from situations they have previously experienced. This practice helps simplify surroundings, keeps teams from having to relearn mundane and redundant strategies, and greatly speeds up the decision process. Humans look for patterns in all the stimuli they experience. This helps to put things in order, chunk information into understandable pieces, and correlate things that look like they belong together. (See **FIGURE 4.2**.)

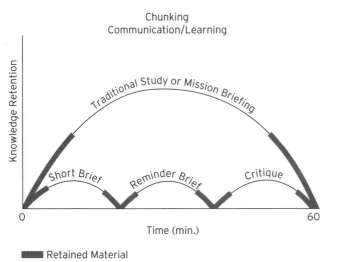

FIGURE 4.2 The practice of regularly evaluating performance (by "chunking" feedback into smaller, more frequent debriefings) allows teams to develop situational awareness, avoid having to relearn strategies, and engage in a more efficient decision process.

These amazing abilities have a few critical drawbacks. Namely, teams might "see" a pattern where none exists and make determinations based on information that only partially fits together. The need to put information into an orderly format is so strong that responders often fill in the missing pieces of an incomplete story using information they recall from similar situations they have faced in the past. Within the team environment, this can lead to serious errors in gaining a collective understanding of a situation. It also helps to explain why each individual team member sees things differently. Because they have not had the same past experience and are not using identical "fill" material to complete the picture in front of them, conflicts can occur. The open communication of CRM is intended to allow team members to respectfully challenge one another when these situations arise.

If one individual sees what they believe is a complete picture, and it differs from another's, it's important to determine why. Analyzing or determining the "why" may not be possible during a time-compressed incident, but it is important to delve into this during the postincident analysis. If team members honestly exchange their views, they might find out exactly where they "inserted" information to complete their picture, and by examining this behavior they are likely to gain a better understanding of what to do next time.

Those with experience understand that the power of recognition-primed decision making comes from the fact that the model does not rely on perfection or absolute accuracy. Instead, plausibility, pragmatic understanding of the situation faced, coherence between team members, the ability to invent solutions, and flexibility form the basis of the critical decision process while under time pressure. This can also be a drawback, particularly when the outcome of a situation is undesirable or tragic. The intuitive decision is difficult to analyze retrospectively because it is nearly impossible to "forget" the outcome while trying to take the point of view the front-line operator had while immersed in the event.

This is important to remember when teaching CRM because those reviewing individual and team performance need to understand that they are looking at the decisions that were made with a mind-set that is substantively different from the mind-set of operators during the emergent event. A critique is primarily analytical, the outcome is known, and a fact set is available for study, whereas the critical decision process is primarily intuitive. The implementation of CRM can wither and die if the organization doesn't understand how decisions made intuitively while under pressure can look terrible during retrospective analysis once the outcome is known. This could cause the organization to place individual blame, which is likely to shut down the open communication process and stifle creative on-scene dialogue. There many examples of these risks.

CASE STUDY 2

Officer Julan Jeffries wondered how it had come down to this. The evening had started as they all do, with routine traffic calls, the occasional alarm response, and a few miscellaneous behavior problems between couples. Now Officer Jeffries stood behind the circle of paramedics who were working to package and transport a 17-year-old male who Officer Jeffries shot just 12 minutes ago.

To say that events had unfolded rapidly would be a gross understatement. Officer Jeffries and his partner, Officer Piper, had pulled up behind the 2002 sport utility vehicle, with its driver and two passengers, on Belmont Street near 32nd Avenue after watching it roll through a stop sign. Jeffries

(continues)

ran the license plates and learned there were no warrants or outstanding violations. He turned on his overhead lights and swung behind the vehicle as it pulled to the curb.

As Officer Jeffries carefully approached the vehicle on the driver's side, Officer Piper started to exit the patrol car. Suddenly, the right front passenger jumped out, ran around the front of the SUV, and pulled something from his waistband. Jeffries immediately drew his service weapon and fired four times, striking the man three times in the chest and once in the right arm. Piper drew her weapon but did not fire. Patrons in an adjacent restaurant dove for cover beneath their tables, and Jeffries withdrew behind the driver's door of his squad car for some protection. Pulling his AR-15 rifle from its mount, he ordered the remaining occupants to stay in the vehicle, with their hands out the window, until his backup arrived.

Once the scene was secure, the paramedics were allowed to treat the passenger. After just a few minutes of resuscitative efforts, the medics on scene pronounced the victim dead, and he was covered to await the investigation team. The "gun," it turned out, was a cell phone.

Officer Jeffries and Officer Piper were experienced, knowledgeable field operators with significant high-fidelity training. (**High-fidelity training**, used by emergency physicians, police officers, paramedics, and fire fighters, is simulation-based, often uses real settings or computer simulators, and is designed to help field operators gain recognition-primed experience in low-frequency, high-risk events.) In the law enforcement world, when someone acts in a threatening manner, the person who reacts slowly may be injured or killed. This was drilled into Jeffries during his high-fidelity training, and he also learned it institutionally after his previous partner was shot in the leg five years earlier while chasing a methamphetamine addict down an alley.

Immediately, people started questioning the officer's decision process. Without seriously considering the officer's context (he had seen a previous partner get shot when he reacted too slowly), the media and some citizen groups started making accusations that the police were not effectively trained, that Officer Jeffries had acted too hastily, and that his decision process was flawed. Unfortunately, this particular police organization chose to suspend the officer and came up with 14 pages of findings related to how officers in similar situations should behave in the future.

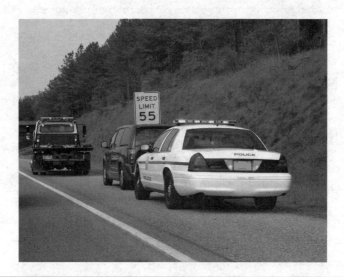

The lesson of Case Study 2 is that critical decisions, whether made by fire fighters, paramedics, or police officers, are made in a dynamic environment. Once the outcome is known, these decisions are easily taken out of context. Individual field operators are held accountable for decisions that they make during time-compressed events, when they have little concrete information and the situation is dynamic and physically dangerous. Retrospectively, the events look simple.

Maintaining context during the evaluation of critical decisions allows an organization to learn from the event while embracing the real-world environment of the field operator. Analyzing how decisions are made and retrospectively applying knowledge of the outcome to refine the field operator's response are important for the development of CRM. Often, high-fidelity training is the only exposure a field operator will get to a high-risk event. By seeking a deeper understanding of how the decision process works on both the individual and team levels, it is possible to develop scenarios that will provide front-line personnel with rich experiences and that challenge their CRM skills.

Summary

Critical decision making takes place in an environment that is dynamic and that can be highly dangerous. Veteran operators remember previously encountered scenarios, weigh the risks and benefits of the immediate alternatives, and choose the best option. Experienced front-line operators evaluate few options because they are typically influenced by what worked well the last time they faced a similar situation. Novices typically recall written protocols and procedures.

CRM is enhanced by a diverse team that understands how decisions are made and that can effectively manage and use conflict. By slowing the decision process in some situations, the team can process more information and can achieve a better outcome.

The next chapter introduces specific concepts related to team behavior and crew resource management. It discusses how teams can manage the flow of information, how they make sense of information presented to them, how they deal with ambiguity, and skills for maintaining situational awareness.

Wrap Up

Ready for Review

- If conflict is well managed, it can be a very healthy attribute in teams. Conflicting viewpoints are a normal part of the decision process during a dynamic situation.
- A good team understands conflict, its role in the decision process, and its importance in vetting alternatives. The key is to keep the dialogue respectful and not to personalize the differences in opinion.
- Conflict brings out the alternatives, emphasizes goals and objectives, and allows the team to come to a shared understanding of what needs to be done.
- When viewing the exact same scene, every person has a slightly different perspective, which is based in part on each person's area of expertise, level of experience, quality of training, ability to recall applicable written procedures, and personal context.
- Any group on an emergency scene shares two significant realities: No one knows exactly how the situation will unfold, and no one knows the outcome.
- Previously experienced situations assist in developing patterns or rules that can be applied in dynamic environments.

Vital Vocabulary

Cognitive control The collection of brain processes that are responsible for planning, cognitive flexibility, abstract thinking, rule acquisition, initiating appropriate actions and inhibiting inappropriate actions, and selecting relevant sensory information.

Conflict Actual or perceived opposition of needs, values, and interests.

High-fidelity training Simulation-based training that often uses real settings or computer simulators and that is designed to help field operators gain recognition-primed experience in low-frequency, high-risk events.

Recognition-primed decision Quick, effective decisions that operators make when faced with complex situations. In this model, the decision maker is assumed to generate a possible course of action, compare it to the constraints imposed by the situation, and select the first course of action that is not rejected.

Rule-based analysis Attempts to capture knowledge of domain experts into expressions that can be evaluated and known as rules. These rules can be compiled into a rule base so that operators can evaluate current working conditions against the rule base and chain rules together until they reach a conclusion.

Assessment in Action

1. Decisions made in a dynamic environment share which of the following characteristics?
   A. Information about the situation is incomplete.
   B. Time is compressed.
   C. Crew stress is high.
   D. All of the above
2. Raecognition-primed decision making:
   A. is a slow methodic process.
   B. encourages adherence to rules.
   C. is based on cues gained from experience.
   D. is not appropriate in emergency situations.
3. CRM emphasizes which aspect of crew behavior during decision making?
   A. The most senior person on the crew makes the decision.
   B. Rule-based decision making is the system that should be used.
   C. Junior members of the crew should not participate.
   D. Dialogue between crew members should occur when there is conflict.
4. Rule-based decisions:
   A. are made using policies and procedures previously established.
   B. should never be used in a dynamic environment.
   C. should always be used in a dynamic environment.
   D. are usually out-of-date and are not reliable.

In-Classroom Activity

Discuss a set of protocols/standard operating procedures (SOPs) and its application in a time-compressed decision-making process. For example, in the opening scenario with the tree-cutting incident, how would a SOP stating "no actions should be taken until qualified electrical power grid personnel are on site" affect the life-saving decisions that need to be made?

5

The Concepts of Crew Resource Management

Objectives

- Describe how a crew can develop a shared understanding.
- Describe the importance of diversity of opinion to crew resource management.
- Describe how to build team expertise and flexibility.
- Describe how to remove boundaries, establish trust, and earn respect.
- Describe how to use an assertive statement.
- Describe the differences between novice and veteran behavior.
- Describe how to maintain situational awareness.
- Describe how to minimize the factors that cause the loss of situational awareness.
- Describe how to improve collective situational awareness by understanding error.
- Describe how to reduce distraction and stay focused.

CASE STUDY 1

Rescue Flight Four, a Bell 430 helicopter, hammered through the hot August day, eating up the miles between its base station in the city center and the rural Cherry River, where fire crews were searching for a lost child who was believed trapped underwater. Paramedic Maria Gomez, sitting up front with Pilot Marty Chase, eyed the towering thunderclouds that appeared to grow in front of them. Frantic radio transmissions could be heard from the scene: Fire fighters in a boat, using an underwater camera, had spotted the little girl and would be deploying divers any moment. Gomez flipped the visor of her helmet up and looked over at Marty, expecting him to comment on the weather. At that very moment, Marty pulled his microphone close to his mouth and said to the medical crew, "I need your full attention here."

Nurse Tom Polk, who was riding in the back of the aircraft preparing medical equipment, turned in his seat and stuck his head into the front compartment. Tom could see the heavy rain falling from the clouds, and he also could hear the ground crews as they prepared to attempt a rescue. The pressure was on.

Marty spoke up, "I can divert around to the west of these squalls, but it will take an extra 10 to 12 minutes. Alternatively, we can turn around and tell the ground crews to transport by ground."

Gomez looked at Polk, who had far more airborne experience. Polk said, "Let's try going around, Marty, and if you see anything at all that makes you worried, abort and we'll let the fire fighters know immediately."

Marty then restated to the crew his intentions. "We're going to try an approach that diverts us to the west. If any of you gets uncomfortable, or if you think it's going to take too long and we should advise them to go by ground, speak up." Gomez gave the ground crews the new updated estimated arrival time, and Marty banked the aircraft to the left. Thankfully, the crew was able to skirt the storm, and 20 minutes after taking off from their hospital base, the big 430 settled onto the grass near a large camping area.

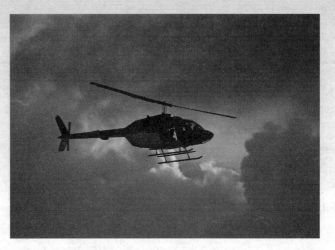

Gomez and Polk with their medical equipment bags stepped from the helicopter moments after it touched down. Both crouched low and hurried toward the group of fire fighters who were working near the bank of the Cherry River. Gomez, who also worked as a fire fighter/paramedic in the city where the aircraft was based, noticed that none of the local fire fighters working next to the river were wearing personal flotation devices (PFDs). She knew that at the agency where she worked, PFDs were standard safety equipment for anyone working near a body of water. Glancing over at the fire department pickup that had towed the boat to the scene, she noted several PFDs stored in the pickup bed. Before she could say anything to the incident commander, however, the little girl was pulled from the water and placed into the boat.

Thirty minutes earlier, three-year-old Susie Bailey had slipped away from her family, who had been seated at a nearby picnic table. After searching for a few minutes, the family called the local fire department, who responded with their water rescue team.

Paramedic Gomez and Nurse Polk started resuscitative efforts the moment Susie was removed from the boat. After they placed a breathing tube in her trachea and started CPR, they moved Susie to the aircraft for the return trip to Samaritan Trauma Center.

As Rescue Flight Four landed on the helipad at Samaritan Trauma Center, the flight crew was met by a team from Samaritan's emergency department.

> During the short flight, Nurse Polk and Paramedic Gomez had been able to restore Susie's pulse, but the little girl had not yet started breathing on her own. With Polk managing the airway and Gomez stabilizing the intravenous lines they had started, Susie was wheeled into the brightly lit trauma bay.
>
> As the flight crew handed off care of their patient, they watched the highly trained physician and nursing team go to work. Even though every movement looked well choreographed, Polk and Gomez could see that Susie's cardiac rhythm was starting to falter. Several minutes went by as the flight crew stood on the side watching a medical resident and the attending pediatric emergency medicine physician continue the resuscitation.
>
> Paramedic Gomez then observed that the patient's abdomen was distended, and she turned to comment about it to Nurse Polk. However, Nurse Polk had left the trauma bay, and the physician team continued to work. Gomez then leaned in and mentioned the distended abdomen to the nurse taking notes. Her concern was that the decrease in ventilatory capacity caused by a distended abdomen could make the child retain carbon dioxide, creating an acidosis that could cause cardiac problems.
>
> However, even after Gomez's comments, the recording nurse remained silent, unwilling to challenge a doctor. After several minutes Paramedic Gomez spoke up and mentioned the distended abdomen to the attending physician, suggesting that decompressing the abdomen might help. A quick assessment by the trauma team revealed a high carbon dioxide level and a low pH. The medical team decompressed the stomach, ventilations became easier, and the cardiac rhythm stabilized. However, Susie died a day later from complications.

Developing a Shared Understanding

Most systems designed for emergency response and care identify safety as their primary objective. High performance, professionalism, and service all take a back seat to the provision of a safe working environment for the front-line operators and a safe experience for the customer. It can be helpful to understand that although safety is (and should always be) the number one priority, emergency response systems will never be completely, inherently safe. Emergency response and care systems exist to provide a service within environments that are often not completely secure, where operators must take action under circumstances that present physical danger, where the human behavior they encounter is poorly understood, and where they face the dynamic development of problems they may have neither the training nor experience to solve.

What usually makes these systems work well is outstanding performance by the operators and constant attention to any situation that may threaten the outcome or the safety of the team. Because no individual is capable of maintaining a constant vigil against errors, and no single person sees all sides of a developing situation, the key to safety during emergent, dynamic situations is leveraging the power of the front-line operators to develop a shared understanding of the goals and of the developing situation. Once a team attains a shared understanding, decision making is more complete, the team can review more alternatives, and safety is enhanced through situational awareness. This shared understanding is accomplished through the use of crew resource management (CRM).

As mentioned in Chapter 4, effective CRM ensures that every member of the team appreciates each of the following key points:
- The exact nature of the problem, its cause, and any confounding or complicating factors
- The skills, strengths, weaknesses, and experience of their fellow team members
- What is likely to happen based on taking no action
- What is likely to happen if the team chooses a specific action

- The desired outcome
- The strategy and tactics that will be used, by whom, and when
- The fact that any member of the team, regardless of rank or experience, can respectfully question the strategy and/or provide additional cues that will help the team gain a better understanding of the situation as it unfolds

Importantly, all team members should know what parts of their system are inherently safe and where the greatest risk lies. They should all be actively engaged in minimizing risk wherever possible while accomplishing the stated objectives.

Consider the flight of Rescue Flight Four in Case Study 1 as an example. During the mission, in several instances operators, regardless of their affiliation, made decisions that could have affected the outcome. Because all emergency scenes contain elements of danger, operators are best served when they communicate well and minimize the number of shortcuts they take during the operation. Front-line operators cannot simply follow rules for every situation they encounter because context is important and not every situation is the same. Typically, written procedures are not sensitive enough to deal with subtle variations in how a situation unfolds, and experienced and trained operators must make well-informed decisions.

Rescue Flight Four's crew faced their first critical decision while en route to the scene of the drowning. Thunderstorms loomed ahead, and such storms pose a danger to in-flight aircraft. In addition, the medical crew keenly understood that transporting the patient by ground would take more than 45 minutes, and Susie's chances of survival under those conditions were slim. Through the use of clear and open communication, the flight crew shared an understanding of the situation:

- They knew the cause of the problem (thunderstorms). They knew about any complicating factors (a reroute would cause a delay).
- They knew the skills, strengths, and weaknesses of their fellow crew members. The pilot knew that Nurse Polk had experience and valued his input on whether a delay or aborting would be prudent. Paramedic Gomez was less experienced than the veteran Polk and she looked to him for a quick analysis of the situation.
- They had an understanding of what would happen if they took no action (they would enter a highly dangerous storm condition).
- They had a shared understanding of what would happen if they continued the flight, but diverted around the storm (they would have a delayed arrival, possibly affecting patient outcome).
- They had a shared understanding of what would happen if they aborted the flight (the patient would have a long ground transport).
- They had a shared understanding of the desired outcome (a short flight for a critical patient, and a safe flight for the helicopter crew).
- They had a shared understanding that any member of the team, regardless of rank or experience, could question their strategy and suggest alternatives (Marty reiterates that anyone with concerns should speak up).

This is effective team communication, and it helps ensure safety for both the crew and their patient. However, it does not guarantee a safe flight, with no complications or adverse outcomes (because nothing can). What it does provide is a comprehensive approach to understanding every known aspect of the situation.

CRM: A Comprehensive Approach

As mentioned in previous chapters, before CRM can be effectively used, there first must be a foundational change in organizational culture. CRM is an effective tool, but improved individual and crew performance comes from using the tool within a working environment that values feedback and constantly works to minimize error. Individuals within such an organization improve because they operate in an atmosphere that provides safe, direct, and respectful feedback on their performance, and they broaden their knowledge and skill base because they assume responsibility for overall team performance. Team performance improves through open communication and the identification of potential tripping points. Issues that might directly affect mission goals and/or personal safety are identified, called to attention, and dealt with.

CRM also focuses on the power of diversity within a team. (See **FIGURE 5.1**.) This diversity is not just associated with cultural or gender viewpoints, but also with the diversity of experience, domain expertise, and technical operating aptitude. **Diversity of opinion** is necessary to avoid groupthink. It is important for leaders to be surrounded with people who will respectfully speak up when they see the need for input.

In addition, the adoption of CRM principles should improve the organizational understanding of attitudes and behaviors. CRM provides an individual understanding of how errors contribute to learning.

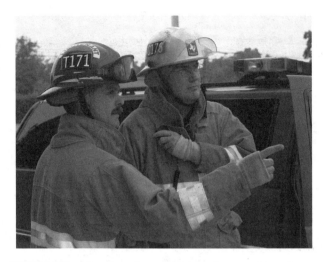

FIGURE 5.1 Diversity of experience and opinions is a powerful asset during an emergency.

It is critical to define just who the crew is in CRM. If CRM focuses on both the outcomes and the safety of the mission, ideally everyone who is involved, regardless of their affiliation, is a member of the crew. This means all personnel engaged in the operation are responsible for ensuring that a shared understanding is exactly that—shared by everyone. This can be exceedingly difficult when crossing different professional domains or when different agencies are involved.

Returning to the banks of the Cherry River, Paramedic Gomez immediately recognized a safety issue when she noticed that the fire fighters operating on the river bank were not wearing any PFDs. As someone who had training in CRM, she knew how to respectfully intervene when she saw a violation of safe operating procedures.

Typically, when a person from one agency must give constructive feedback to a member of another agency, the person preparing to give feedback evaluates several factors prior to engaging. Gomez may have asked herself these questions:

- Is there a reason for them trading accuracy (safety) for speed? It would have only taken a moment to put on the PFDs. She may look for a reason to validate their behavior.
- Do they look like they would take feedback, even if it is respectful? Gomez may determine that their level of anxiety and agitation over the age of the patient and their initial inability to find her could cause them to react badly to her suggestion. Who is she, anyway, to tell them about the value of PFDs?
- Are there other things of a more urgent nature that need her attention? Gomez may do her own "trading" of options, deciding that taking action to prepare for Susie's arrival onshore is more important than warning the fire fighters about their lack of PFDs.

Regardless of how Gomez formed her decision, it can be assumed that if she said nothing to the fire fighters, there was no shared understanding of the danger they put themselves in. They may have known, on some level, that not wearing PFDs was a risk (after all, the agency provides them for a reason). It can also be assumed that if one of them fell into the river and drowned, at least one operator on scene would have said, "I knew that would happen."

This simple statement should help drive the input of a team member. If everyone is striving for high performance and safety within dangerous and ambiguous environments, then each team member carries a responsibility for helping to provide a shared understanding of the scene, for contributing to the collective situational awareness. Whether the input is acted upon is not necessarily each responder's responsibility, but team members should always attempt to engage if they see that without intervention, something could happen that would adversely affect team members or the outcome.

In the case of the fire fighters with no PFDs, Gomez should have said something to the on-scene crew. And if it wasn't possible for her to engage them on scene, then she should have followed up afterward with the incident commander to gain collective situational awareness of danger points.

The Role of the Team Leader

It is important to clarify what CRM is not designed for. CRM is not team decision making. Every team needs a leader, and the leader is tasked with carefully listening to input, evaluating the options, leading any discussion if there is conflict, and ultimately making the decision on which course of action is appropriate. The team provides open, honest, respectful input, but the leader decides on the action plan.

CASE STUDY 2

Captain Mario Morando tried turning around in the narrow space between the long commercial kitchen countertop on his left and the large gas stoves on his right. Every time he moved, his self-contained breathing apparatus (SCBA) air bottle clanged into one obstruction or the other. All he could see in front of him were the bottoms of Fire Fighter Jack Davis's boots, and the 1¾-in. (44-mm) hose line that snaked by his side. He knew from the familiar noises he heard that Jack had the nozzle wide open, trying to make headway against the heavy flames blowing above their head. When Morando looked over his shoulder, he could barely see the helmet and facemask of Apparatus Operator Dave Brown, who had one hand on Morando's boot and the other on the hose line, helping to drag it forward. Morando knew that Fire Fighter Weaver was behind Brown, and he started to worry about their ability to retreat if necessary.

The Casa Lupita Mexican Restaurant was a popular place. The bar was large and multilevel, and it opened to a large food court. Morando knew from experience (both from tours and as a patron of the establishment) that the roof was supported by several graceful steel arches.

At 4:20 AM when Brown had turned the corner from the highway onto Hall Boulevard, Morando could already see the glow from the fire. Minutes later, as his crew pulled into the parking lot, he saw that heavy flames had breached the huge stained glass window that anchored one end of the bar. Captain Morando's engine was the second due, and his crew was told to pull an attack line into the kitchen at the rear and fight the fire from there. After his crew pulled the line, Morando gathered them together at the entrance to the kitchen. They quickly checked each other's personal protection, verified their air levels, and prepared to enter. Morando turned to his crew and said, "Jack's got the nozzle, I'll follow with the thermal imager. Dave, you're pulling line behind us and you'll have the irons. Weaver, you block the doors behind us, grab the short pike, and make sure we don't pass something that's burning. This'll be a direct attack. ... Everyone OK with that? Also, this building has a steel arch roof supporting tile. It's heavy. I want everyone to keep their eyes peeled." Everyone nodded agreement except for Weaver, who spoke up: "Cap, you want a second line by the door? I can go grab one. ... " Morando looked back into the lot and saw that other engines were arriving. He told Weaver, "No thanks," and they proceeded into the kitchen.

Now Morando found himself in a highly uncomfortable situation. He knew they were pouring 250 gallons a minute onto the fire from the kitchen door, and it did not appear to be darkening. Instead, the heat level continued to increase. Morando guessed they had been inside the kitchen for at least 15 minutes. The fire had likely been burning long before they were called, having only become visible after it broke through the windows of the bar. Morando also knew that the building had a heavy clay tile roof. He radioed the incident commander that his crew was going to retreat from the kitchen. They were pulling out. He reached forward and grabbed Davis's boot, giving it a few hard jerks backward to get his attention.

Fire Fighter Davis immediately wedged the nozzle under his right leg and partially turned to face his captain. "What're we doing, Cap? Why pull out? I think if we go a few more minutes, we'll have it licked." Behind him, Fire Fighter

Weaver also yelled updates to his captain: "It's pretty hot back here, Cap. Also, we've got a lot more hose line if you need it." Brown suggested Morando take another look with the thermal imager. As Morando rolled to his right to get a better look toward the ceiling, he peered through the viewfinder and was surprised at how much the temperature had risen since they entered.

Morando rolled back onto his hands and knees, clipped the thermal imager to his belt strap, and simply started backing down the long narrow hallway, pulling the hose (and Jack) with him. As the crew reached the small vestibule near the kitchen door, they heard a loud cracking sound. Dropping the hose line, they heard Battalion Chief Dennis King over their radios: "Emergency Traffic, all units abandon the building. Repeat, abandon the building."

As Morando's crew cleared the door, he double-checked to make sure everyone was accounted for. Almost immediately, the roof of the building over the bar area caved in, showering the parking lot with broken glass, stucco, and roof tiles. Captain Morando and his crew quickly moved back and were directed to continue fighting the fire in defensive positions.

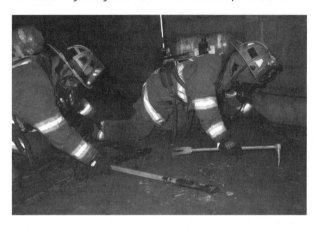

Respectful Feedback

The degree of respect provided in *respectful feedback* depends on the makeup of the crew, the length of time they have worked together, and their operating context. Deference to rank is common in hierarchical systems such as the fire department or police department, but so is the friendly banter often found among personnel who feel almost like family members. It's important that leaders of teams set expectations about how they want feedback, and they must address privately any concerns when a team member acts in a manner that shows disrespect.

In the case of the Casa Lupita fire, Captain Morando demonstrated several different aspects of CRM in action. First, upon the initial fire attack, he outlined the team roles and made sure that each crew member had a shared understanding of the chosen strategy. Next, he asked for input ("Everyone OK with that?"). He also developed a shared understanding of a particular risk associated with that building, reminding everyone to stay alert.

Once the fire started to intensify, the decision process became compressed. In such situations, there is little time to discuss alternatives, and because everyone has a different viewpoint, there are bound to be disagreements on what course of action to take. Morando was an experienced fire officer, and he was uncomfortable. He had a knowledge of the building, an understanding of what happens to metal arch trusses when they are impinged by fire, and a sense of how long his crew had been in the building. He followed suggestions from his crew (double-checking with the thermal imager), listened to their input (if the fire fighter farthest away from the flame front notices an increase in heat, that's a powerful signal), and also acted decisively when necessary.

The stressors placed on the crew leader can be powerful. Consider what could have occurred if the crew of Rescue Flight Four let their emotions determine their actions. After all, they had a three-year-old who was in critical condition and a group of fire fighters on the ground counting on their arrival. Captain Morando at Casa Lupita could also have let the pressure of his veteran fire fighter get to him.

The weight of decision making can be particularly heavy when the team leader is younger than other crew members and when the leader has less field expertise or experience than team members do. In cases where leaders are new, they must remind themselves of the overriding objective: Take no risk that need not be taken and keep the crew safe. The decision is theirs, not the team's.

Building Team Expertise and Flexibility

Within high-performance teams, regular use of CRM to gain a shared understanding continually improves performance. Specifically, when teams practice communication techniques that are designed to share understanding, it provides opportunities to build team discipline, broaden the knowledge base of individual team members, and remove hierarchal boundaries to learning. Additionally, leaders can establish trust and respect, reduce the chance for error caused by distraction, and encourage collective situational awareness.

Team leaders should know that each member has his or her role and domain expertise. Because CRM is an interactive and participative process, formal roles must be clearly communicated. It's important for each team member to understand how every member's role brings value and supports the team objectives. However, team leaders also are responsible for determining levels of experience within the group, outlining expectations, and openly asking for constructive input.

Increasing the knowledge base of team members is a core duty of team leaders because every team member brings particular domain expertise and must accomplish a specific task. Because of their backgrounds and experience, team members each have unique ways of viewing problems. Good team leaders encourage members to understand each other's roles and responsibilities and to pay particular attention to each other's areas of weakness as well as expertise. By "cross-pollinating," members learn who to turn to when specific problems arise. They also develop a basic understanding of what they should look for when any single team member reaches the point of task saturation, which is defined as too much input and not enough time to process all the information.

By sharing domain experience with each other, members become more apt to speak out when someone becomes overwhelmed or believes a fellow team member may have missed a cue that is important to their individual task and the team's collective success.

Removing Boundaries and Establishing Trust and Respect

Good teams develop a level of trust that goes beyond technical expertise. They actually come to understand the importance of collectively solving problems and value the diversity of opinions within the team. Diverse opinions, in any team, lead to some level of conflict. In this context, conflict is not bad. Instead, the success or failure of a team is often predicated on how the team manages conflict and whether they are able to benefit from conflict by using it to outline strategic differences.

The trust developed within a team using CRM is based predominantly on the core value of respect. Every team member, when confronting an idea, action, order, or behavior, must exhibit respect for their fellow members, regardless of their rank, position within the team, or level of expertise. Consider the following.

CASE STUDY 3

As Medic Two turned into the stadium parking lot, the crew saw a crowd by the entrance to the football field waving at them frantically. Paramedic Larry Ierulli, a veteran of 22 years, turned to his partner, Hannah Glaser, and said, "I have a feeling this is a bad one." Hannah carefully steered the ambulance through the crowded entrance and onto the track surrounding the field. A knot of people stood on the nearby 30-yard line, watching three team officials work over the football player, 17-year-old Casey Waters. His helmet had been removed, and it appeared to Larry that one of the men was attempting to ventilate the player using a bag-valve-mask (BVM) device. "Told you so," said Larry to no one in particular.

Hannah and Larry grabbed their equipment bags, a cardiac monitor, and spinal immobilization equipment and ran over to the downed player. The small crowd of people moved aside, allowing them to see that lineman Casey Waters was unconscious, unresponsive, and occasionally combative. The man holding the BVM device told Larry that he was Dr. Josephson and that he was the team physician. He ordered Larry and Hannah to place a cervical collar on Casey and to move him to the ambulance.

Larry knew that Casey needed an advanced airway procedure immediately to survive. Casey had definitely suffered a serious head injury, and a quick check of his pulse showed bradycardia, the slow heart rate that often precedes cardiac arrest when there is serious respiratory compromise. Larry also knew that Dr. Josephson was probably not a trained emergency physician, or he would have recognized the condition himself and ordered a different course of action.

Rather than antagonize Dr. Josephson, Larry turned to Hannah and told her to prepare the airway kit for a rapid-sequence induction. They would have to medically paralyze Casey and put a tube down his trachea. Knowing Dr. Josephson might object, he turned to the physician and said, "Doctor, I see you've started using a BVM. Thank you for noticing he has a serious airway problem. Please continue your ventilations, and I'm certain you agree that Casey needs immediate intubation. Also, we'll use paralytics, which will keep him still and help us immobilize him in case of a head or neck injury."

After rapidly starting an intravenous line and administering the paralytic medications, Larry quickly intubated the football player. After securing the tube, he handed the ventilation bag to the physician and asked, "Dr. Josephson, would you be so kind as to ventilate Casey for a few minutes while we prepare him for transport? Also, we are considering transporting him to the nearest trauma center, what do you think?" Dr. Josephson agreed, and the crew of Medic Two moved Casey to the ambulance.

After the crew delivered Casey to the trauma center, Hannah asked Larry why he let the physician continue helping them with patient care when he clearly didn't know how to manage an emergent airway. Larry replied that embarrassing Dr. Josephson in front of his team would serve no purpose and would likely lead to a situation where the doctor would need to defend his authority.

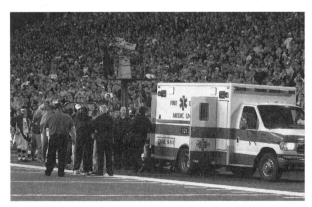

CASE STUDY 4

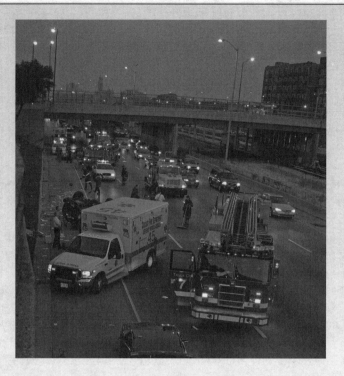

Apparatus Operator Miranda Hopper pulled Engine 23 carefully into the inside lane of Interstate 5, positioning the pumper at an angle so that it completely blocked the lane and provided her crew with some protection from the oncoming traffic. In front of her, she could see four cars had spun into each other. The middle two looked significantly damaged, and the occupants were still inside.

Her officer, Lieutenant Fred Charles, stepped off Engine 23 onto the icy roadway. This was the engine's sixth call on Interstate 5 in the last three hours, and the snowstorm had started getting worse. Fred was cranky. The police had not yet closed the nearby on-ramp, and traffic continued to attempt to enter the freeway even though they could see the severe conditions. Fred hated freeway calls and had suffered two close calls over the past year since he had been assigned to Station 23. In one instance, a driver had plowed right into the back step of the fire engine as it sat in the traffic lane. Had it not been for good positioning of the apparatus, Fred and his crew could have been critically injured or killed.

Miranda was intimidated by Lieutenant Charles. He was experienced, vocal, and generally impatient. However, after the entire crew received training in CRM, he had openly asked his crew for input on several occasions, which surprised and pleased her. Tonight, after positioning the fire engine, she noted that traffic in the middle lane was still coming fairly close to the crew as they worked the scene. Miranda approached Lieutenant Charles and asked if she could reposition the big rig so that both lanes were blocked, providing them more of a safety buffer. Lieutenant Charles, stomping around the scene, told her, "No, I need you up with the Triage Officer."

> Politely persisting, Miranda told Fred that she would hustle right up there immediately afterward, but that she thought moving the engine was necessary. Lieutenant Charles suddenly turned to her and snapped, "What part of 'no' don't you understand?" Without further comment, Miranda walked up to assist the fire fighter performing triage.

Learning to disagree respectfully without being disagreeable is a practiced skill. So is accepting critical input without voicing or exhibiting displeasure at the sender of the message. An individual's response to input determines the quality and amount of feedback that person receives from team members. If a story is created that a team leader or a particular domain expert becomes defensive or "prickly" when given feedback that he or she might construe as critical of a decision, or if internal repercussions exist that are associated with challenging someone with more rank or expertise, the effectiveness of CRM is significantly blunted. It is likely that Miranda will never again give feedback to Lieutenant Charles, regardless of how important the situation. In the case of Dr. Josephson, however, Larry set the stage for continued communication by quickly determining how to avoid friction.

In emergency situations, communication should flow freely, but members should know where the final decision lies. Once the entire team has assessed situational factors, the leader still must make a decision. Initial decisions are only the beginning of the CRM process. After every decision comes a course of action, and a good leader immediately solicits input related to the effectiveness of the previous action or decision.

Choosing a Method of Engagement

Many in the fire service and EMS believe that challenging the decisions of a superior undermines the authority of the paramilitary system. How does a team member approach a superior and tell him or her that a foul-up is brewing? The answer lies in the team member being an advocate for his or her position while at the same time understanding the leader's position. One of the most effective methods for advocating a position is by using an **assertive statement**. The five parts of an assertive statement are as follows:

- Using an opening statement that addresses the person by name ("Chuck," "Captain," "Chief")
- Stating the concern as an owned emotion ("I think we are heading for a problem.")
- Stating the problem as the team member sees it ("It looks like that building is getting ready to flash.")
- Offering a solution ("I think we should evacuate the interior crews right now.")
- Obtaining agreement ("Do you agree?")

Using advocacy helps promote situational awareness and improves understanding. When fire fighters, paramedics, police officers, dispatchers, and other public safety workers use advocacy, they rightfully believe that they are in charge of the situation and become more willing to meet goals and objectives.

Team Behaviors: The Differences between Novices and Veterans

A key factor in great teamwork in pressure situations is the ability of team members to filter sensory input and differentiate mere distractions from important cues. In a recent study at Tualatin Valley Fire and Rescue (TVF&R) in Portland, Oregon, EMS and operations leaders were interested in determining how veterans filtered information and whether information that veterans filtered out could retrospectively be understood as missed important cues. In particular, the study showed that there was a noticeable difference in the number of decision points recognized by veteran officers and paramedics versus novices.

First, through interviews with industry professionals, the department defined the terms *novice* and *veteran*. Rather than simply using time in grade or longevity, veterans were determined to have had exposure to 2000 incidents, of which they had to be Paramedic in Charge (PIC) or Incident Commander (IC) on a minimum of 200. The researchers used the descriptions of 42 fire incidents and 165 medical incidents that all had rich detail available including video, audio, photos, and written reports to present as scenarios to cohesive teams of fire fighter paramedics. Team leaders who had been designated either PIC (medical incidents) or IC (fire or rescue incidents) were asked to note points in the scenarios in which decisions had to be made, either by them as the leader or by another team member.

Novices recognized decisions on fire scenes three times for every one decision point noted by a veteran, and on medical incidents the disparity was even greater, with a 4:1 ratio of novice decision points to veteran. Most telling, the novices noticed decision points more often when there were multiple distractions present in the scenario (radio transmissions, cell phone calls, and face-to-face discussions occurring at once) or when the situation seemed somewhat ambiguous (no policy or protocol specifically provided guidance). Veterans, however, simply ignored most of the distractions or made efforts to minimize those they felt were intrusive and not helpful (turned down some radio channels, silenced the cell phone, and rolled up the windows in the command vehicle or cut short the one-on-one discussions).

Because they knew the outcomes, the researchers knew which cues were important and which ones were mere distractions. A common mistake in postincident analysis is to develop hindsight bias and "know" what operators should have looked for. In this study, it was helpful to know so that the decisions could be evaluated in context, as a whole incident, and not as separate decision points. Observers were to note when it appeared the team had lost their situational awareness. When this occurred, novices most commonly halted all actions and scanned for situational cues. More than 70 percent of the time, they then became distracted by cues they had earlier dismissed as unimportant, and they also were less effective in getting their team to help them filter information.

The conclusion of the study was that novices had a more difficult time keeping up with critical information flow from complex scenes, and that they could quickly fall behind the incident if they lost situational awareness, even temporarily. This was largely a result of the novices' tendency to become more tentative in their decision making after having made a situational error. Veterans, on the other hand, tended to shrug off the error and to quickly reprioritize the incoming cues with their team to ensure that they were not missing something important, all the while maintaining control over the scene that continued to develop in front of them.

What this means is that team leaders need to be aware of how novice members of the team process incoming information. Novices pay more attention to cues than veterans do, see things in greater detail, and are more apt to try and associate current team strategies with organizational policies and procedures. This can provide value in that novice operators often "see" detail, particularly related to safe operating practices, that seasoned veterans might overlook.

Team Behaviors: Keys to Maintaining Situational Awareness

Situational awareness has three primary components: cognitive awareness of the surroundings and how individuals are supposed to interact with the surroundings, the reality of the situation, and individual perceptions of the situation. Situational awareness is an internal active evaluation process that goes on constantly, much like size-up. Operators update their situational awareness constantly by observing their surroundings, evaluating their options, and communicating with those around them.

The dynamic, fluid emergencies that fire fighters, EMS, and law enforcement personnel respond to require that they maintain the absolute highest state of alertness and attention at all times. Because emergency workers are human and subject to the same human frailties as the rest of the general population, loss of situational awareness does occur. This loss of situational awareness is common when they perform routine tasks in familiar surroundings. It is a penalty they pay as they gain expertise and experience. As emergency workers gain skill, they often pay less attention to the mundane details of everyday operations. But these details can become important as a situation becomes complex and teams look for cause-and-effect solutions. Consider the scenario in Case Study 5.

CASE STUDY 5

After Paul LeSage had been a flight paramedic for more than six years, he faced a gruesome and startling example of how ignoring the mundane in the field of emergency care can lead to death. It had become somewhat of a joke among the flight paramedics that a few of the pilots always repeated the exact same warning every time the crew exited the aircraft: "Watch the tail rotor," the pilots would say without fail. Every time, on hundreds of flights, the same warning: "Watch the tail rotor." Medics would respond, "Yeah, I know, it hurts."

Then came a day when Paul and his flight crew responded to a call at a popular ski resort, where they were using helicopters to film a ski movie. The flight crew was to transport a patient who reportedly had severe head trauma. Upon arrival, they found their patient had a large head wound and massive brain injury. He was the pilot of one of the film helicopters, had years of experience, and he had walked into his own tail rotor. Suddenly, the constant reminder of the obvious had more meaning. Regardless of how experienced you are, it only takes a second, a minor lapse in attention or judgment, to cause a catastrophe.

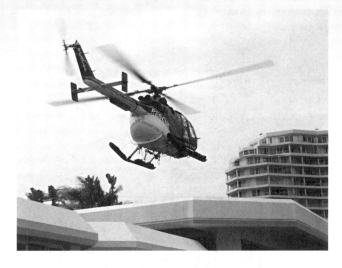

Maintaining situational awareness is a skill that can be taught, regardless of the domain. Essentially, the following behaviors help teams maintain situational awareness:

- Being suspicious: Leaders need not be paranoid, but truly curious of anything that could interfere with a smooth-running operation. This means challenging routine events and habits. They should ask themselves and their team questions about why they are doing what they are doing. The questions should require specific answers and the leader should be satisfied that everyone has gained an understanding of the objectives.
- Ask team members, "What can go wrong?": This should be a challenge question: Given their domain expertise and their job, how do they view the operation? What, in their eyes, poses the biggest risk? What is the smallest risk? What would happen if either of those things occurred? How would the team regain control of the situation?
- Reducing the need for **cognitive processing**: Cognitive processing is a scientific term for the process of thinking. Leaders should use checklists when appropriate to minimize the chance of missing a step while multitasking. They should ask the veterans about how seriously they are taking incoming cues related to a developing situation. What are they filtering out, and why? What do the novices think? Are there policies that are relevant? Leaders should use their team completely, rely on their abilities, and encourage open communication and a closed feedback loop, which means ensuring that questions and actions receive a response. Practices related to reducing cognitive load can have a sharp edge, however. Making checklists for critical tasks while on scene is a great idea, but leaders should not lose sight of the steps themselves, and why each one is important. This is accomplished through regular training and challenging teams as mentioned earlier by asking, "If I missed a step, what could go wrong?"

- Reducing the opportunity for unnecessary distraction: This can be tough because one individual's distraction is another's important cue related to the developing situation. Leaders should ask their team about certain reductions before taking action. For example, before turning down the volume of a specific radio channel or closing the window or the doors to the command center, leaders should ask out loud if the action will help to reduce that particular distraction. They might be surprised when someone speaks out and says, "Don't turn down that radio, I'm waiting for an important message from the safety officer."
- Openly discussing performance-shaping criteria for the team: Leaders should ask team members whether they have experience with a particular task. Are they comfortable? Do they need assistance? Also, team members should call attention to factors that may appear obvious, such as stress, fatigue, noise, and workload. When a team member calls attention to these factors, he or she gives the group permission to acknowledge how their own performance may be affected.
- Regularly stating the primary mission of the team: Once distracted, a team can head off in a tangential direction that allows a critical loss of situational awareness. This is directly tied to the concept of "Who's flying the plane?" Pilots know that regardless of the number of distractions, their primary mission is still to fly the plane. In a medical context, this can be stated as: "Let's bag the patient, ladies and gentlemen. A, B, C, let's not forget the basics," or on a fire scene as, "Make deliberate and safe moves, everyone. The building is a loss, let's stay safe and protect the exposures."

CASE STUDY 6

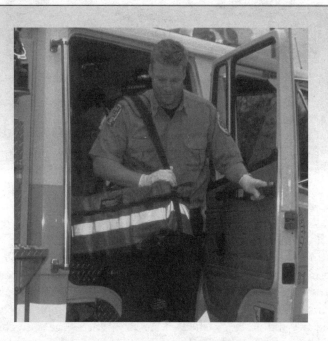

Fire Fighter/Paramedics Vic McCallister and Rob Cooper worked on Rescue 4 in the Palisades neighborhood, which is known in the city of 1.5 million people as the local "knife and gun club." Both prided themselves on being good at their jobs, particularly when it came to managing trauma. Rescue 4 was located at Fire Station 22, along with Engine and Ladder Truck 22. Vic and Rob enjoyed the camaraderie they felt among the 10 people on their shift, and they thought that being at the busiest station in the city helped them stay sharp.

Vic was relatively new to the team, with 3 years experience, and Rob was an old veteran who had been on Rescue 4 for 16 years. When Vic arrived, he introduced some new concepts to the team. One of his ideas was to place breakaway security tabs on the zippers of some of their little used medical kits to reduce the amount of time they spent checking inventory every morning. These tabs, which held the zippers closed until you snapped them off, had a space where the crew member performing inventory would note his initials and the date he checked the compartment in the bag. These tags also indicated a date in the future when the first item inside that particular compartment reached its expiration point.

Team members at Station 4 thought the idea was brilliant. They were very busy and rarely completed an inventory without interruption. The idea spread to other stations and soon it became an unwritten practice within the organization. There were no policies developed on how to accomplish securing inventory, but the agency willingly purchased the security tags and distributed them through their supply system.

Eighteen months later, at 10:34 PM on August 16, 2007, Rescue 4 and Engine 22 responded with a local ambulance company to the residence of Eddie Grant. Eddie reported that his two-year-old daughter Moisha had been running a fever, and when his wife went in the bedroom to check on her, Moisha was unresponsive and not breathing. That night, both McCallister and Cooper were working Rescue 4.

Upon their arrival, Vic and Rob grabbed their medical gear and ran up the stairs to the Grants' second-floor apartment. Engine 22 was close behind. Rob stated he would take "PIC" (Paramedic in Charge) and began barking orders at the team of rescuers. Vic grabbed the airway kit and started providing Moisha with respiratory support. Rob told Lieutenant Welch, a paramedic on Engine 22, to get the pediatric kit opened and prepare for an intraosseous (IO) infusion (a needle that is placed into bone marrow, primarily in a patient's leg).

Lieutenant Welch pulled the pediatric kit up into their working area and recognized that all the compartments were locked closed with tabs on the zippers. More important, he had no idea which compartment held the critically needed IV equipment, so he asked Vic McCallister. Vic was also unable to tell him, and so Lieutenant Welch popped open every tab and started rooting through the kit, frantically looking for the needed equipment. In the anxious moments that followed, later testimony would bring out the fact that someone on scene finally turned the kit upside down and dumped out the contents in a pile.

Once the IO equipment was located, the crew had difficulty putting it together, not because they hadn't been trained to do so, but because this was a high-risk, low-frequency task that they were performing under pressure and simultaneously with other tasks.

Moisha Grant died, but not because of the actions on scene. According to the coroner's inquest, she was dead for at least 30 minutes prior to the arrival of Rescue 4. During a comprehensive postincident analysis, it was determined that one of the system problems was the slow development of a practice that allowed situational awareness to erode. Placing security tags on some equipment meant that the pediatric bag was only opened every six months or so (pediatric cardiac arrest calls, even in a busy system, are

(continues)

> thankfully few and far between). Additionally, because the crew that opens the tags and does inventory once every six months is one of three shift rotations at each station, a situation was created where some paramedics may not ever see the equipment, where it is located, or how it goes together over an 18-month period. This was not an individual problem but a system problem that went unseen by everyone involved.

Maintaining awareness and high reliability requires regularly checking assumptions. If the crew in Case Study 6 had asked one of the critical questions posed earlier ("What could go wrong if we implement this practice?"), they might have collectively determined that the risks were not worth the benefits.

Although this is clearly hindsight bias, it helps define those daily practices that can work against teams later if they stop paying close attention to the details, in other words, if team members stop being suspicious or curious about any potential outcome of our actions.

Minimizing Factors That Cause Loss of Situational Awareness

Following are several of the more common factors that lead to distraction or loss of awareness. Operators must remain vigilant for the appearance of these factors and take action to arrest their influence in intense, dynamically developing situations:

- Ambiguous statements or situations: Team members who make ambiguous statements are usually trying to make sense of their surroundings or the situation. They often see something that doesn't fit, and their statements are designed to express concern without overtly stating that they don't know what's going on. Team leaders need to pay attention to random, ambiguous statements and "close the loop" by asking for clarification. "What specifically is your concern? What do you see that is bothering you?" These types of questions help provide a collective understanding within the team. Often other members see the same ambiguous cues, but they remain quiet, fearful that they are the only ones who "don't get it." Ambiguity in situations must also be brought out and clearly stated. If the team doesn't understand why a particular thing is happening, it helps to bring that forward and ask for suggestions: "I haven't seen this situation before, has anyone dealt with something similar? Who might we ask for assistance? What do you think is going on here?" Questions like these help bring a shared understanding of the problem. Sometimes one team member completely understands what is happening and assumes that everyone else does, too. Assumptions can be dangerous. If the statement or situation appears ambiguous, work to provide clarity.
- Failure to deal with distraction: Dealing with distraction is an art form that is developed over time. As shown earlier in the TVF&R study, veterans had an uncanny ability to manage distraction, and novices were often unsure what was an important cue and what needed to be ignored. Team leaders need to regularly ask about the removal of distracting elements. Will removing certain items reduce their overall situational awareness or contribute to the team's ability to concentrate on the most important tasks and objectives? Studies have shown that teams that get distracted have a difficult time regaining situational awareness. Guard against this by watching for distracting elements (leaders must ask other team members what is distracting them) and openly discussing how to close out these elements. (See **FIGURE 5.2**.)
- Fixation on a single objective or a nonperforming strategy: Fixation is common when there are multiple distractions. One method humans use to improve performance is to consciously block out things that are not directly tied to our primary objective. In firefighting, this is often called the "moth to flame" effect, when inexperienced fire fighters initiate an aggressive, offensive fire attack without considering appropriate risk-benefit tactics. In EMS, it takes the form of emergency care providers paying so much attention to one procedure that they ignore other important cues. For example, paramedics have been known to become fixated on the patient's ECG tracing without carefully looking to see whether the patient's

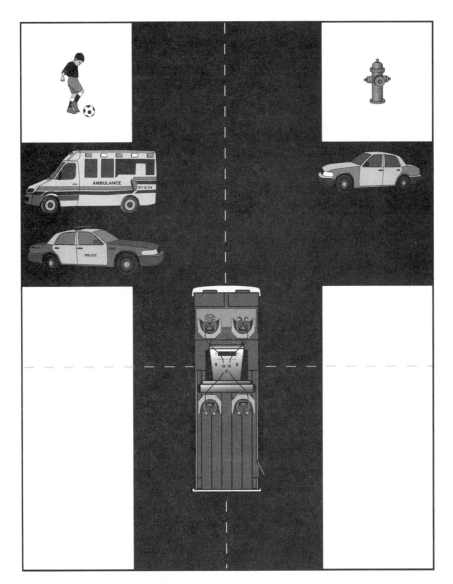

FIGURE 5.2 Maintaining a sterile cab is one method of dealing with distraction during emergency response. Sensory inputs must be managed appropriately in order for the driver and officer to maintain a focus on safety and the mission objective. Cutting down on nonessential conversation removes distraction and allows all team members to be aware of things in their environment that could compromise safety.

symptoms are congruent with what is shown on the monitor. In one case, paramedics were preparing to defibrillate a patient because the monitor indicated what appeared to be ventricular fibrillation, but in reality the cables had come loose. Fixation on a nonperforming strategy is also a danger and can cause loss of situational awareness. This typically occurs when a team leader becomes defensive when his or her strategy is challenged. The leader believes that the chosen strategy isn't working because the team isn't working hard enough. The leader believes that changing focus or adopting another strategy is an indication of weakness or indecisiveness.

- Task overload: This is related to the success strategy mentioned earlier, where effective teams work to reduce their cognitive processing. It is often said, if something needs to be done, give the job to a busy person. But this is a dangerous tactic in a high-performance team. Leaders need to balance workload between team members whenever possible. At times, it is impossible to stay ahead of the information coming in and the tasks that need to be accomplished. When this occurs, effective team leaders purposefully slow the momentum of the team ever so slightly and allow team members to prioritize. Taking a moment to prioritize tasks as a team leads to shared understanding of consequences.

- Complacency or a misplaced sense of comfort: Few people come to work wanting to be labeled as complacent. Yet, in accident reports, complacency is often listed as a cause. Complacency itself is not an accident cause, it is an effect. Complacency is the effect of an organizational sense of comfort with certain routine procedures or practices. These procedures or practices are done so often and within the same environment that operators often lose sight of their importance. This is especially evident with safety practices that are allowed to go unchecked, such as seat belt use, appropriate glove use, and use of personal protective equipment. In the case of Rescue Flight Four discussed earlier in this chapter, Paramedic Gomez recognized that the fire fighters along the riverbank were not wearing PFDs. Had one of them fallen in and drowned, the cause would likely have been listed as complacency. But again, complacent behavior is the effect of an organization ignoring the small elements that make up the collective safety cushion at a scene. It is possible to remove several layers of that cushion and often suffer no ill effects. Once these behaviors become an accepted practice, individuals cannot be faulted, but the organization must take responsibility for not emphasizing the importance of paying attention to the "small things" that lead to complacent behavior and bad outcomes.
- Implementing an improper procedure, or not following a good one: When is it appropriate to deviate from standing operating guidelines? As stated earlier, policies cannot address all the subtle differences that occur in emergency situations. Experienced operators must determine the best method for implementing procedures that are designed to help them achieve a good outcome. However, they must do this in a dynamic environment where the procedures often become simply background context, meaning the procedures are often general guidelines that operators have deviated from slightly on numerous occasions with no adverse outcome. Next, the new deviations become the general practice, and then when some adverse outcome happens people are held accountable to the written rules. Good team leaders consider this, and they understand those situations when a deviation is necessary to achieve the objective. They also understand and discuss the risk-benefit ratio of doing things differently so that the entire team has a shared understanding of the risks. Failure to do so can lead to a loss of collective situational awareness, particularly because novices rely on procedures to guide them while veterans use experience and intuition.
- Failure to resolve or properly manage conflicts or conflicting conditions: Team leaders need to pay close attention to managing conflict. As stated earlier, conflict is a normal, helpful part of collective problem solving if it is managed correctly. This means ensuring people are heard, closing the communication loop, and maintaining respect among the team members. If there are conflicting conditions, team members must call attention to the conflicts so that shared understanding of the priorities and goals develops.

In the study discussed earlier, researchers found that when veterans lost situational awareness, they tended to choose a fallback position and quickly rebuild an action plan based on their new information. They were distracted or slowed by unimportant cues only 15 percent of the time, and they typically actively engaged their team in scanning for new inputs that would help them clarify the situation.

The study clearly demonstrates that veterans are more effective at reducing distraction, and that distraction tends to pull team members away from the original objectives and often causes a collective loss of situational awareness. Although there are many ways to reduce distraction, most are specific to the type of environment the operator is immersed in during work. For example, fire commanders have multiple sources of incoming stimuli and other critical factors that influence their decision process. A noncomprehensive list includes, at a minimum, the following:

- The type of structure burning, and the dangers or challenges it poses
- The immediate risks (people, other structures, or environment.)
- The immediate strategy that should be employed, and a secondary strategy

In addition, they may have to deal with the following:
- Dispatch radio frequency
- Tactical radio frequencies, with multiple companies, divisions, and groups
- An emergency frequency (mayday channel)
- A base and/or staging frequency
- Citizens and others (utilities, police, etc.) coming up to the command vehicle with questions, comments, input

- Cellular phone calls from command officers or others
- Media
- Fire personnel approaching for face-to-face communications

They must manage all this in the face of a dynamically changing environment, where decisions often need to be modified based on expected versus actual outcomes.

Improving Collective Situational Awareness by Understanding Error

Situational awareness is the extent to which an individual's understanding of the immediate environment mirrors reality. If it is considered that each person's reality is framed by his or her individual understanding of the current situation, relative experience, and responsibility to act, it becomes clear that situational awareness is a very personal thing. Typically, once the incident is over and all the necessary information to evaluate performance is available, it is possible to, "see" what the operators "should have" seen or experienced during the incident.

So, how does CRM improve something so personal as situational awareness? Primarily, it forces the team to act in a manner where everyone gains a shared understanding of the goal, is aware of incoming cues within their own spheres of influence and expertise, recognizes information that may be vital to the outcome, and communicates this information to the entire team effectively on a regular basis. (More practical applications are addressed in the next chapter.)

In addition, collective situational awareness can be improved as the team learns more about how errors occur within teams. Understanding how an error begins and grows into a larger, more complex challenge sheds some light on how team members can mitigate these lapses in the early stage.

Errors are typically classified as individual errors or team errors. These classifications are further divided into categories that help emphasize the need for clear communication and collective situational awareness: Errors are either *dependent* or *independent*. **Dependent individual errors** occur when some of the information available to the operator is incorrect, incomplete, or absent. **Independent individual errors** occur when an operator has the correct information, but makes a mistake in cognitively processing the information or experiences task saturation. Team members who recognize that another member may be making an independent error have the responsibility to speak up and point out the lapse or mistake. Alternatively, particularly if the operator making the error is task saturated, the team member may decide to take action to ensure that the team does not fail in its mission.

If a team member identifies a gap in the information that the team needs to make a decision, it is important for that team member to indicate where the gap exists or to point out the cues that the team is missing. By pointing out when dependent and independent errors are being made, team members can help each other and the team become more aware of how they fill in gaps between information they receive and when to step in and assist fellow team members at critical times during an event.

Team members practicing CRM, then, have several responsibilities: They must each individually learn to watch carefully for missed cues and potential individual errors. They must detect the occurrence of such errors, or they have no chance to correct them.

Once an error is detected, recovery from the error or outcome depends on whether team members bring the error to the attention of the group. When a team member detects an error but does not indicate it to the remainder of the team, there is a good chance that the team will execute actions based on the erroneous assumptions.

When a team member detects an error and indicates it to the rest of the team, the team must then correct the error. This is the most critical point of the decision process. The team leader is responsible for acknowledging that the team member indicated an error (or a potential error based on a stated course of action) and must then decide whether the current action plan is still warranted or modifications are needed. At this point, leaders must be most aware of their innate need to reduce cognitive dissonance. Good team leaders don't consider these indications to be a personal attack on their knowledge, performance, or situational awareness, but instead use them to question the status quo and challenge shared beliefs about the current situation.

Reducing Distraction and Staying Focused

Reducing sensory input can help operators stay focused on the task(s) at hand. Obviously, this can have a significant downside. What sensory input should be reduced? How should operators determine what is an immediate need or communication, and what can wait?

It can be helpful to look at three properties that can cause distraction and a loss of situational awareness: information load, variety of information, and ambiguous information. Information load can be understood as a mixture of the quantity, variety, and ambiguity of data streaming into the team. As the load increases, team members are each affected differently, but at some point each person begins to engage filters to manage the information. The first behavior a team member demonstrates to filter information is usually omission, where the individual consciously or unconsciously simply stops paying attention to one source of stimuli, such as a radio channel. Team leaders need to understand this particular behavior because the cues that team members ignore may be critical to a successful outcome.

An increase in the variety of information that is presented to the team is common and can cause distraction. Team members may be engaged with everything from immediate tactical objectives to determining long-term logistical needs, or the tactics themselves may require a broad understanding of several different disciplines (for example, a fire involving hazardous materials and patients that have been exposed). This is where a diverse team shines. When members have wide-ranging experience and good communication skills, they can better manage interactively complex situations.

Ambiguous information is another distracting factor. When operators have difficulty understanding the information or there is dissonance between what they believe should be happening and what is actually occurring, they take more time to process the information. More of their attention is drawn to issues that don't fall neatly into any category with which they are familiar, meaning the time they spend making sense of ambiguity affects how many other information cues they can receive and understand. For example, consider the failure of a piece of equipment on scene. In one such case, medics watched the cardiac monitor as their patient apparently flipped from one serious cardiac rhythm into another. The patient, however, appeared to be tolerating it well. The medics were so focused on resolving the ambiguity between the patient's apparent condition and the condition as it appeared on the monitor that they failed to realize that the monitor was repeating the same pattern of cardiac rhythms over and over again, each one for a set period of time. The machine was set in "training mode," which ran prescribed cardiac rhythms one right after another for interpretation purposes and was not reading the patient's actual cardiac output.

As operators speed up their information processing, they also tend to make assumptions that fit into their schema, the framework they are building to solve the current problem. Because these assumptions can lead to unsafe actions, the leader should remind team members to question the incoming information. By doing this, the entire team "understands" the same things, and suppositions about the situation are minimized.

Language and how team members use words can cause additional problems with assumptions because they don't always know when they should clarify statements and they don't always recognize errors until after they have been made. This is one reason why so many agencies no longer use "10-codes" to communicate over the radio because a "10-22" for one agency could mean something entirely different to another agency responding to the same scene. Even clear text is not free of errors and assumptions of meaning. In one case in California, police officers attempting to apprehend a criminal asked a group of Marines working with them to provide "cover." To the police officers, *cover* meant that the Marines would take up positions and prepare to fire if necessary. To the Marines, *cover* meant laying down cover fire. The difference was startling, to say the least.

Perceptions can be perilous in the dynamic and risky environment of the emergency provider. The late sociologist Robert K. Merton provided another clear example of how language affects individual perceptions. Merton described an experiment in which people were told they were in the presence of objects described as "gasoline drums." The people exercised great care: Smoking was prohibited and they followed safety procedures carefully. However, when another group of people were presented with what were described as "empty gasoline drums," their behavior tended to be far more careless, even though empty drums, with their large vapor space, are more dangerous than full drums.

A final argument for working to reduce distraction and interruption is associated with internal human physiologic responses. Certain actions or thought processes trigger activity in the human autonomic nervous system. As the autonomic nervous system responds to a "threat," people lose some capacity to process information and think rationally. The extent to which rational thought process degrades is debatable, but it most certainly depends on how individuals interpret the stimulus and whether they believe it is something that requires immediate attention.

This physiologic response, then, reduces the number of external cues operators pick up about the current situation. Solving a crisis places an urgency on the decision-making process, time becomes compressed, and teams may completely ignore cues or stimuli that would have otherwise seemed relevant. (See **FIGURE 5.3**.)

Emergency service providers, like soldiers, have developed methods to deal with situations where arousal increases to a point where individual and team performance breaks down. The normal and appropriate response is to practice complex situations in a high-fidelity training environment. Some of the most successful

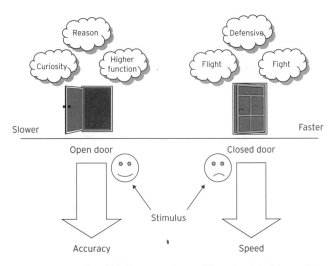

FIGURE 5.3 Emotional intelligence and recognition-primed decision making.

models introduce distraction, multiple cues, ambiguous information, and time pressure during a critical training operation so that the team (and individuals) can practice the same types of tasks over and over. This can help shield teams from performance degradation during times of critical stress; however, skills must be practiced on a regular basis to ensure high reliability.

Instituting Situational Awareness Within a Culture

In 2005, the staff at Henderson Fire, while attending the National Association of EMS Physicians (NAEMSP) conference, learned of a study from San Diego that involved rapid sequence intubation. Alarmingly, the report indicated that 57 percent of patients were desaturating during facilitated intubation (the patient's oxygen levels dropped dangerously low during attempts at placing the airway tube). Facilitated intubation is when an emergency worker places an endotracheal tube or advanced airway using only sedatives or anesthetics and without paralyzing the patient.

Henderson Fire had always benchmarked the successful control of an airway much like the rest of the nation did, by successful placement of the endotracheal tube. When they compared local data to the study, new issues emerged. They found that to achieve a high completion rate, it was apparent that multiple attempts at intubation were necessary. Henderson then examined the effects these multiple attempts had on patients and found results similar to the San Diego study: Henderson's patients were desaturating during the multiple attempts at intubation.

The Henderson EMS staff completed a task analysis, which demonstrated that human error was inevitable given the multiple tasks required of a paramedic performing a facilitated intubation. Because CRM was just making its way into the organization, the staff developed an EMS task standard using a military model for facilitated endotracheal intubation. (See **FIGURE 5.4**.)

For an EMS provider, the decision to actively paralyze a patient, decrease the patient's level of consciousness, and control the airway is a high-risk, low-frequency event. The situation is typically dynamic and time compressed, and decisions can be more complicated when difficult airway criteria are identified, such as short necks, small mouth openings, suspected obstruction, blood in the airway, combative patients, or the need for cervical immobilization.

Henderson developed a facilitated intubation task standard using CRM concepts of task allocation, an open communication model, clarification of the mission, and collective situational awareness. They use a specific checklist to train personnel on their roles and tasks, with the goal being standardization of techniques and reduction of error.

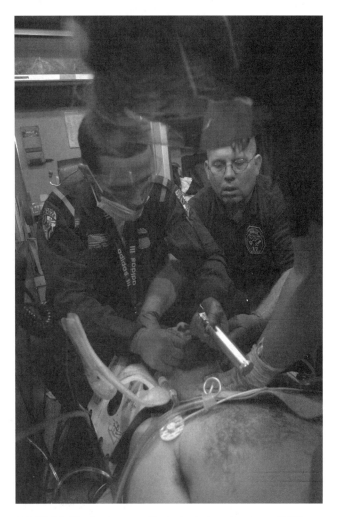

FIGURE 5.4 The development of task standards centered on a CRM theme help improve the safety profile of a high-risk, low-frequency event.

CHAPTER 5: The Concepts of Crew Resource Management

Task standards divide responsibilities among individuals and teams, allowing for effective completion. Henderson created three specific positions for a facilitated intubation team, each with unique responsibilities to ensure a safe and efficient procedure. Medical staff communicated to the organization a clear mission with the goal of providing an advanced airway with adequate ventilation. Individual paramedics understood that the new task-oriented procedure was focused on patient care and that the entire crew was responsible for the success of the process.

The communication model built into the task standard uses a closed feedback loop to ensure coherence and to maximize situational awareness. The paramedic responsible for performing the intubation receives constant feedback regarding pulse oximetry results and is asked to verbally acknowledge the oximetry reading during the procedure. Redundancy is purposefully built into the task-oriented procedure; for example, in the absence of accurate pulse oximetry, the patient's heart rate and elapsed procedure time are secondary parameters used to maintain collective team situational awareness. Collective situational awareness is a key component in that the team is constantly made aware of the oxygenation status of the patient so that they maintain an accurate perception of the events as they unfold in real time.

One common error that leads to a loss of situational awareness during facilitated intubation is the tendency of individual operators to ignore or disregard information that may be given out of context. In the past, random statements by team members, such as "the patient is experiencing bradycardia," or "you've been in the airway for more than 30 seconds" were consciously ignored or simply not heard by a paramedic fixated on that single critical component of the mission, passing the tube through the cords.

In this case, a critical evaluation by the organization and the development of task standards centered on a CRM theme helped to improve the safety profile of a high-risk, low-frequency event. This use of CRM when performing critical airway interventions in the field is an example of best practices by an EMS organization.

Summary

To understand how crew resource management can be used most effectively, teams must understand many important concepts. Team members must gain a shared understanding and acknowledge that the "crew" may well extend beyond the boundaries of their own jurisdiction.

By taking a comprehensive approach that values expertise and flexibility and incorporates trust and respect, teams can build cohesiveness. Importantly, a foundation of these values can be laid earlier when the organization deals with the power of story and the damage that can be done if team members don't understand how to manage half-truths that become stories related to performance.

In an open communication model, team members practice proper forms of interpersonal engagement and use respectful advocacy. In this context, the greatest value comes from knowledge that no one individual is as effective as a team when the team is openly and honestly communicating.

Certain key behaviors are associated with maintaining and losing situational awareness. One of the greatest values of an open communication model such as CRM is that the team can effectively gain and maintain a collective situational awareness. In addition, by calling attention to the performance-shaping factors described in this chapter, teams are alerted when they recognize signs that situational awareness could be eroding.

By reducing the propensity for individual errors and practicing techniques to minimize distraction, team effectiveness grows. These are learned behaviors that take time to master, and they require attention to detail by the team leader.

The next chapter discusses implementing a model for crew resource management. Now that a comprehensive foundation is laid and the effects organizational culture are understood, factors in the decision process, and specific behaviors have on implementing a successful program, it is possible to focus on the mechanics of the process.

Wrap Up

Ready for Review

- Emergency response and care systems exist to provide a service in environments that are often not completely secure and where operators must take action under circumstances that present physical danger, where the human behavior they encounter is poorly understood, and where they face the dynamic development of problems they may have neither the training nor experience to solve.
- With a shared understanding of the goals of the mission and the developing situation, the team can make more complete decisions, review more alternatives, and enhance safety through situational awareness. Teams gain shared understanding through the use of crew resource management.
- CRM focuses on both the outcomes and the safety of the mission. Ideally, everyone involved, regardless of their affiliation, is a member of the "crew."
- Every team needs a leader, and the leader is tasked with carefully listening to input, evaluating the options, leading any discussion if there is conflict, and ultimately making the decision on which course of action is appropriate.
- The trust developed in a team that uses CRM is based on the core value of respect. Every team member, when confronting an idea, action, order, or behavior, must exhibit respect for fellow team members, regardless of rank, position within the team, or level of expertise.
- Recovery from errors and the outcomes of situations are dependent on whether team members bring pertinent information to the attention of the group. When an error is detected but not communicated to other members of the team, there is a good chance that actions based on erroneous assumptions will be executed.

Vital Vocabulary

Assertive statement A communication that consists of five parts that enable respectful communication between crew members: (1) an opening statement that uses the addressed person's name, (2) a statement of concern as an owned emotion, (3) a statement of the problem as you see it, (4) the offer of a solution, and (5) obtaining agreement.

Cognitive processing A scientific term for the process of thinking.

Dependent individual errors Errors that occur when some of the information available to the operator is incorrect, incomplete, or absent.

Diversity of opinion When people respectfully speak their opinions when they can offer input gained from diverse experiences, domain expertise, and technical operating aptitudes.

Independent individual errors Errors that occur when an operator has the correct information but makes a mistake in cognitively processing the information or is "task saturated."

Assessment in Action

1. Situational awareness is:
   A. individually focused only.
   B. only important in the early stages of an incident.
   C. an individual and crew responsibility.
   D. easy to keep track of.
2. Crew communication in an emergency environment:
   A. is best served by a paramilitary structure.
   B. benefits from assertive statements.
   C. should be free of conflict.
   D. has no use for diversity.
3. The use of checklists and procedures:
   A. reduces cognitive processing during periods of high stress.
   B. indicates a crew weakness in remembering important things.
   C. should be delegated to junior team members.
   D. is not really very helpful.
4. Primary decisions at an emergency scene should include:
   A. saving lives and property at all costs.
   B. minimizing risk and considering crew safety.

C. deferring to group decisions.
D. the use of policy.

In-Classroom Activity

Role-play the opening scenario in which the fire fighters did not use PFDs during a water rescue to demonstrate effective team communication. One role player assumes the position of a battalion chief as IC of the incident, and another role player is a department member who tries to convince the chief to use the PFDs for crew safety.

Remember to use the five parts of an assertive statement:
- An opening statement that uses the addressed person's name ("Chief")
- Statement of your concern as an owned emotion ("I think we are heading for a problem.")
- Statement of the problem as you see it ("The river is running pretty swiftly.")
- Offer of a solution ("I think we should have the crew wear PFDs.")
- Obtaining agreement ("Do you agree?")

Understanding and Implementing Crew Resource Management

Objectives

- Describe how to work in an open communications model.
- Describe how a team member uses inquiry to question an action or behavior that is incongruent with his or her own situational understanding.
- Describe how advocacy allows team members to respectfully question authority.
- Describe how conflict resolution is accomplished in a learning environment.
- Describe how the team leader guides his or her crew toward making a decision.
- Describe how team members "observe and critique" in order to evaluate a decision with respect to initially stated mission goals.
- Describe the process of discussing options, after a thorough assessment of a team's work has been conducted.

CASE STUDY 1

Scenario A
In a large California city, Engine 38 turned onto Bay View Boulevard with its siren blaring. Fire Fighter Andrea Collins looked across the cab at Fire Fighter Ian Ainoa and noticed that he had not fastened his seat belt. She wondered whether to say something to him. Ian was far more experienced than she was and had been working the busy Engine 38 for seven years. Andrea was a "newbie," and this was her first shift working at the busiest and most decorated station in the department.

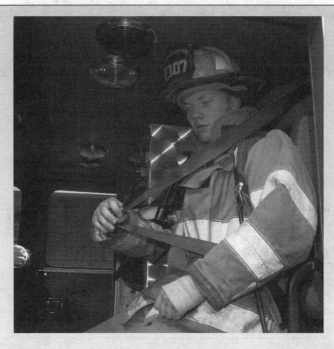

Scenario B

Paramedics Gill Pryor and Mandy Humphrey, working for an urban EMS program in Florida, arrived on scene at Crescent Bay Park, where a 26-year-old woman lay unconscious on the boat dock. Patient Karli Kumar had just been pulled off of a ski boat. Fifteen minutes earlier, she had been struck by another boat while water skiing, and she had suffered a serious head injury. Gill noted that the local fire service was already on scene, and they had started preparing to intubate Karli using paralytic medications. As Gill walked up to the patient's side, the fire medic handed Gill a syringe and said "Push the meds. We are ready with the tube." Gill cleaned off the intravenous port and started administering the medication, all the while wondering what exactly was in the syringe.

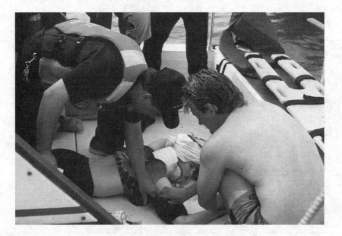

Scenario C

Captain Ronald Goldhaber walked the one block from where his crew had parked their ladder truck to the scene of the fire in a suburban Oregon town. Three stores at the east end of the 10-year-old strip mall were fully involved, with fire pushing out the large front windows. The next exposure was a large jewelry store, and Goldhaber's four-person crew from Ladder 7 had just been ordered to vertically ventilate that particular store. Goldhaber noted that the fire had not yet penetrated the wall separating this store from its neighbors, but there was a considerable amount of black smoke pushing hard from under the front eaves. Captain Goldhaber turned to his most experienced fire fighter, Ted Hackman, and asked him what he thought of the order they had just been given. In the postincident investigative notes, Goldhaber reported that Fire Fighter Hackman had simply rolled his eyes and said nothing. In those same notes, Hackman said that he "knew this was a bad situation," but didn't say anything because "I'm just the fire fighter."

After Ladder 7 climbed onto the roof from the rear of the building, the truss structures in the involved stores failed, pulling the wall of the jewelry store down and subsequently collapsing the jewelry store roof. Miraculously, the roof failed in a rearward direction, and the crew from Ladder 7 literally slid into the parking lot with minor injuries.

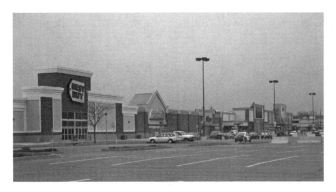

Working with an Open Communication Model: The Circle of Success

Each of the stories in Case Study 1 represents a missed opportunity for shared understanding. Previous chapters discuss why individuals feel inhibited from communicating openly and the types of organizational cultures that negatively affect efforts to gain a shared understanding and high reliability. In this chapter, it is assumed that the ground work has been laid for open communication: The foundation of a just culture is in place, all personnel understand their responsibility for gaining a shared understanding, and the system is ready to provide education and active training on methods of communication.

A crew resource management (CRM) program encompasses a range of competencies, skills, and behaviors, including situational awareness, problem solving, decision making, teamwork, leadership, followership, and self-awareness. None of these refer to the technical proficiencies that team members must also know, such as starting an IV, operating a hose line, doing a surgical procedure, and tying a knot. The cognitive and interpersonal capabilities of CRM crew members must develop and be practiced like any technical skill.

Because CRM skills focus primarily on team members understanding and interpreting their own behavior and that of others, these skills should be learned in an environment with an experiential focus. Practice that includes visual, audible, and tactile interactive team function should be a primary goal of CRM training. In an experiential environment, successful learning has occurred when team members can evaluate their past behavior in a given circumstance and develop personal tools that allow them to be more effective in future, similar situations.

The typical CRM model contains several key elements, all of which are integral to gaining a shared understanding in a culture of learning and mutual respect. These elements are *inquiry*, *advocacy*, *conflict resolution*, *decision*, *observe and critique*, and *discuss options*. In a typical incident, these elements are used in a seamless communication process. Once practiced in this process, the players often do not consciously walk through each step; instead, they use the process automatically, as part of the fabric of an open communication model that allows a shared understanding among team members.

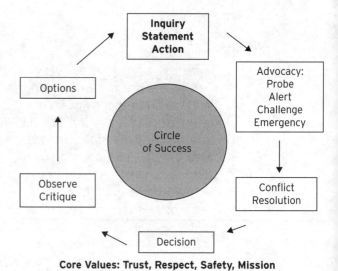

Core Values: Trust, Respect, Safety, Mission

FIGURE 6.1 Inquiry is the first step in the CRM circle of success.

Inquiry

The first step in the CRM circle of success is inquiry. (See **FIGURE 6.1**.) This initial phase is when one or more team members are given a mission *objective*, when someone (typically the leader) makes a *statement* or gives an *order*, or when a team member first recognizes a *behavior* or *action* that might appear incongruent with his or her own situational understanding. An inquiry typically comes across in one of the following forms:

- A statement by a team member or the leader: "This is our objective, and this is plan A."
- An order from someone superior in rank or experience: "Give 50 mg of Benadryl IM" or "Advance a line to the second floor."
- An action: A team member, leader or otherwise, performs an action that draws the attention of other team members.
- A behavior: A team member exhibits behavior perceived as inappropriate for the circumstances.

A statement is declarative. If a statement is made by a superior or someone with more experience or expertise than the receiver, the receiver often misconstrues the statement as an order or a demand. However, it is important for team members to understand that statements are simply declarations of fact or observation and that they can still be questioned.

Factors Affecting Inquiry: Coherence and Sense Making

Two of the most common errors made at the inquiry stage in the CRM process result from miscommunication associated with coherence and sense making.

Coherence

<u>Coherence</u> is associated with how well the receiver understands the message. Coherence is possible when the truth of a situation aligns with phrases, propositions, or beliefs presented by a sender. In some cases, coherence is "asymmetrical" in that the sender means one thing and the receiver hears another because the sender may be using jargon or terminology that is either unfamiliar to the receiver or that has one meaning to the sender and another to the receiver. Consider the following case study as an example.

CASE STUDY 2

Engine 65 of the West Metro Fire Department was called to a working residential structure fire as an automatic aid company to the city of Freeport. As Engine 65 arrived at 1024 Palatine Drive, they noted that two engines and a ladder truck were already on scene, a hydrant was taken, and smoke banked across the street in front of them. The officer reported his arrival to the incident commander, a battalion chief from Freeport Fire. The incident commander acknowledged the arrival of Engine 65 and told them to "stand by" for a few minutes, which they did, waiting in their apparatus for an order.

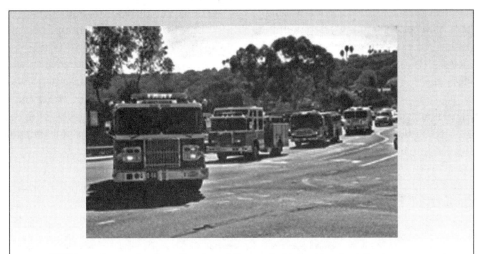

Within a few minutes, Engine 65 was told by the incident commander to "pack up." No further order was given, and the crew from Engine 65 departed the scene, switching to the dispatch frequency and reporting their return. Shortly after they started to return to quarters, dispatch asked them why they were returning. "We were told to pack up and return," stated the officer. The dispatcher told Engine 65 that the incident commander needed them back at the scene. Once they arrived back at the fire, Engine 65 was assigned as the rapid intervention team (RIT).

After the fire, the incident commander was upset about their departure, but when the crew from Engine 65 explained their behavior, he admitted that in Freeport, the term *pack up* meant "don your self-contained breathing apparatus." At West Metro, *pack up* meant leave the scene.

This is a clear example of a coherence problem: The incident commander used terminology that had one meaning for the incident commander and another meaning for the engine company.

Coherence can also be a problem when different agencies use different signals, procedures, or shortcuts (sometimes this occurs even within the same organization). A medic might be asked, for instance, to "give 10 of Benadryl." Did the sender mean 10 milligrams or 10 milliliters? In most cases, the difference in meaning is significant and needs to be clarified. Another example of this might involve an incident commander at a residential fire who has ordered the hose line from the hydrant to the pumper be charged with water. The pumper operator blows his air horn twice, signaling the fire fighter one block away at the hydrant to turn on the water flow. To the incident commander's amazement, two firefighting crews immediately evacuate the building. They are on the fire scene from a different agency that provided automatic aid, and to them, two blasts on an air horn mean "abandon the building."

The best way to deal with terminology coherence issues is for team members to practice repeating back what they think they heard, or what they understand to be correct, not exactly what the person said. "I understand you want 10 milliliters of Benadryl, or 50 milligrams. Is that correct?" For procedural differences (such as the air horn example or the use of "10-codes" that mean different things to different people), it is best in advance of any incident to collaborate with various agencies to standardize regional practices and procedures, particularly those related to safety.

Sense Making

The second phenomenon that often occurs during the inquiry phase is **sense making**, which is a team member's ability or attempt to make sense of an ambiguous situation. Sense making is different from problem solving. When problem solving, the issue that needs to be resolved must first be identified, and then it is necessary to work through options to arrive at a resolution. Sense making, however, occurs when individuals are unsure of what they are experiencing. It is what happens when expectations don't match up with reality, or when individuals experience something that is completely foreign to them.

Individuals in teams, particularly leaders and veterans, must pay close attention when their fellow team members are trying to make sense of a situation. Sense making is a universal experience with both veteran and novice operators, but the novices are more likely to be confused by what they see and make statements based on their fear of the unknown. This is simply because veterans operate in a recognition-primed mode because they have already seen and experienced a similar event. Veteran field operators use **recognition-primed decision making**. Instead of considering many different options, or mentally evaluating the myriad of written procedures and protocols related to a situation, veterans act based on what worked best for them in the past in similar situations. They *recognize* the situation and are *primed* to act in a certain way based on a previous successful (or unsuccessful) outcome. This typically occurs very quickly, while the novice is still evaluating alternatives.

> ### CASE STUDY 3
>
> Probationary Fire Fighter/Paramedic Justin Leach dropped the medical kits at the door to the bedroom and entered behind the other three members of his crew. There on the bed lay the 22-year-old shooting victim. They had received reports of two victims, but Justin could see only the one woman.
>
> As his crew moved the patient to the floor, Justin commented, "I've never seen this much blood." His crew calmly commenced resuscitation efforts, placing an airway, and moving a backboard into the room to prepare the patient for transport to a trauma center. During the resuscitation, as Justin prepared to intubate the patient, he again commented, "This is more blood than I've ever seen."

Justin's paramedic field training officer, Apparatus Operator Gus Lee, recognized what was happening: Justin was sense making, or trying to determine whether what he was seeing and experiencing was "normal and expected," given the situation. Had a veteran team member made the same statements, Gus would have taken them much more seriously. He knew that he needed to support his "probie," by remaining calm and performing his job. He also had to check his own bias ("It's a probie mistake…") to ensure that the amount of blood was indeed consistent for only one victim.

One of the easiest ways to determine during the inquiry phase whether a team member is trying to make sense of a situation is to listen carefully to everyone's comments as the situation unfolds. In the emergency medical services (EMS), fire, and police worlds, what might appear to veterans to be random statements are very typically signals of extreme discomfort. For example, during initial flight paramedic training a probie might comment to the pilot that the rotor blades "sure seem close to those trees" during a landing sequence. This type of statement demonstrates discomfort and unfamiliarity.

Team members, especially leaders, must listen carefully for these types of statements because such statements may be the first sign that something is, indeed, seriously going wrong. The veteran may be so immersed in the situation that he or she has tuned out additional stimuli. The method for dealing with sense-making comments during the inquiry phase of CRM is for the leader to ask for clarification: "What specifically are you concerned about?" Good teams do not allow seemingly random comments to go unanswered or unchallenged. Inquiries, comments, statements, orders, and behaviors all require feedback to validate them or to allow the team to assume a collective understanding of the events as they are perceived by everyone present.

Good practices during the inquiry phase include aggressive listening skills, allowing an environment where respectful commentary is accepted, and carefully intervening to ensure that the question is heard correctly.

Advocacy

In many typical CRM structures, the second step in the communication loop is labeled *advocacy*. (See **FIGURE 6.2**.) However, *advocacy* does little to actually describe the process that occurs when a team member feels dissonance related to something he or she has heard or seen in the inquiry phase. Questioning authority, either hierarchical or expert, is a daunting task. During this step, it is crucial for team members to understand that there are *two*

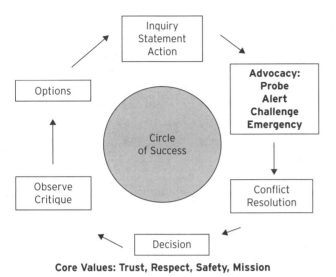

FIGURE 6.2 Advocacy occurs when a team member voices his or her opinion regarding the inquiry at hand.

methods for approving of an action or statement they see or hear, and only *one* method for providing a challenge. The two methods of providing approval for the actions or statements of others are to verbally state understanding and agreement, and to voice no objection at all.

The second method of indicating approval, saying nothing, is all too common—and too commonly misused, as becomes apparent during postincident analyses. During critiques, team members might wonder how much understanding was truly shared at the incident. For example, a team member will state that he or she had a concern, or "knew" something was going to happen, but the person typically has a reason for not speaking up. Leaders are often astonished when they hear this. How could their team member have sandbagged them? Why didn't the person voice an opinion? When team members do not speak up, leaders assume everyone approves after they have asked for input and no one voices an objection.

When this occurs, it is critically important for leaders to step back from their feelings and bruised ego. Instead, they need to be very curious—curious about what kept the individual from participating, curious about the organizational culture, and curious about any verbal or nonverbal cues they send when someone challenges the status quo.

The following case is an instructive example of these behaviors.

CASE STUDY 4

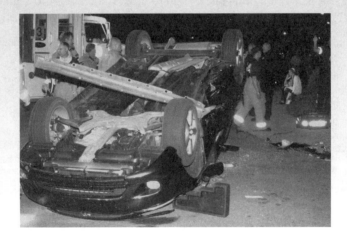

The crew from Advanced Life Support (ALS) Engine 35 arrived on scene at the rollover motor vehicle accident to find the 32-year-old male driver had been ejected into a nearby ditch. After quickly stabilizing his cervical spine, the crew began a procedure to secure his airway known as rapid sequence induction (RSI). This is a high-risk, low-frequency procedure that involves administering powerful paralytic agents to the patient and then inserting a breathing tube into the trachea. Many steps need to be done in a particular sequence, and the crew of Engine 35 was using a prescribed checklist. At some point in the call, the department's well-known and talented EMS chief

(continues)

arrived on scene to provide assistance. The EMS chief drew up one of the induction medications, followed procedure by verbalizing the expiration date and dose twice, and handed the syringe to one of the fire fighter/paramedics, who paused, looked carefully at the syringe, and then proceeded to give the medication. The patient was successfully intubated and transferred to a nearby trauma center for further treatment.

During the postincident critique, the fire fighter/paramedic approached the EMS chief and inquired, "Did you know that the syringe you gave me held only one-half of the recommended dose of the drug?" The EMS chief responded by asking, "Why didn't you speak up and say something?" The answer can be guessed by anyone who has worked within a hierarchical system: "Well, because you are the EMS chief, and I assumed you knew what you were doing."

The EMS chief was surprised. The organization had conducted CRM training, he was seen as an open, approachable person, and there was a viable self-reporting system in place with no corrective action applied for clinical errors. However, when he decided to be curious instead of defensive, he understood that the fire fighter/paramedic had less than two years on the job and had only interacted with the EMS chief a few times over that period. In addition, the EMS chief did not directly ask for input when he handed the syringe to his subordinate (i.e., he did not ask the fire fighter/paramedic to verify the dose). Because the fire fighter/paramedic was not familiar with the chief, and because he was not asked in the team environment to validate the chief's action, he simply made the assumption that the chief must know something that he didn't. Maybe they had changed the dose recently. Why take the risk of looking like he didn't know that? What if the chief were correct? What if the dose was really wrong—how would the chief react?

Such communication and collaboration issues occur regardless of how teams approach CRM. No matter how open the learning environment is, there will always be obstacles, real or perceived, that keep people from speaking up. The high-reliability organization consistently challenges those assumptions and looks for methods to minimize the potential for miscommunication.

PACE

One method that is gaining some recognition was developed for airline crews so that they could effectively challenge seasoned captains. Instead of advocacy, it is called PACE. (See **FIGURE 6.3**.)

The acronym PACE describes a series of actions that team members can take to make better sense of what they see and hear from their leader and other operators:

- **P**robe for better understanding (the sense-making phase).
- **A**lert the leader of any concerns or abnormalities.

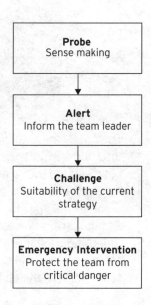

FIGURE 6.3 PACE.

- **C**hallenge the suitability of a current action or strategy if the probe and alert don't appear to be changing the course of action.
- **E**mergency intervention if there is critical danger and the team continues on a course that will cause harm.

The following sections describe each of these steps in more detail.

Probe

A successful probe by a team member is a clear communication that identifies the person who is being asked the question, respects the individual, and is direct enough to be understood. Ambiguous statements addressed to the entire team are not considered effective probes. For example, in the previous case study, if the fire fighter/paramedic had turned to the group at large and asked, "Anyone recall the dose of Etomidate?" this would violate the tenants of a good probing question. First, it is not directed at anyone in particular; therefore, no one has a responsibility to answer, and the question may remain unresolved. Second, it is disrespectful. "How dare he openly challenge my understanding of the dosage!" would be an understandable response from the EMS chief. In addition, there is no way for the EMS chief to recover his dignity and thus there is a greater chance he will become defensive.

A good probe in that case would have been for the fire fighter/paramedic to ask the EMS chief specifically, "Chief, the dose I am familiar with is *XX* milligrams. This is *YY* milligrams. Is this the correct dose, or should we double it?" The advantages of this type of communication are numerous: It is focused and directed—the chief knows someone is asking him for input; and it is respectful and very specific. There is no question or ambiguity about what type of information the fire fighter/paramedic needs to continue with the task.

Additionally, leaders must emphasize that the ability to probe productively is an artful undertaking. It is not typically something that can be conducted effectively while "inside" the emergency. In other words, building trust early, being reliable, and ensuring that the other team members know their best interests are being kept in mind help establish the credibility that is necessary during an event.

Alert

The **alert** phase can be done independently of a probe or after a probe. If the team member recognizes that a course of action appears inappropriate, then there is no need for the sense-making or probing phase. Instead, the team member moves directly to alerting, which is simply and clearly stating what the team member is seeing or experiencing that he or she believes can compromise the mission or objective. Again, this needs to be done respectfully and clearly. The output of a successful team, particularly in maintaining highly reliable performance, is nearly always greater than the effects of individual crew members who are not working in concert with each other. If everyone involved in operations has been trained in CRM principles and there is a shared understanding, clearly there is a safer environment for both the patient (customer) and the crew.

Consider the following case of a dispatcher contributing to a successful fire outcome by using the alerting technique.

CASE STUDY 5

As the fire on Mountain Road continued to grow, Battalion Chief Doug Andersen, the incident commander, knew he was facing a losing battle. It was just past 3:00 AM, and the 14,000 square foot (1300.1 m²) Georgian Colonial home on 15 acres of land was burning to the ground. There simply wasn't enough water for the amount of fire, and he was now worried that the radiant heat would overcome their efforts at protecting a large horse barn adjacent to the home. Because this home was just outside the city limits, no fire hydrants were available and water tender shuttles were bringing in all water. Even with eight tenders, Chief Andersen could only manage a constant flow of about 1000 GPM (63.1 L/sec), meaning he had to shut down direct fire attack and concentrate on a defensive approach.

In the meantime, the Lincoln County Communications Center (LCCC) had just completed sending a full complement of fire apparatus to Chief Andersen's call for a third alarm. Inside the LCCC, Fire Dispatcher Aaron Meade pulled up the aerial maps associated with the area. Because they

(continues)

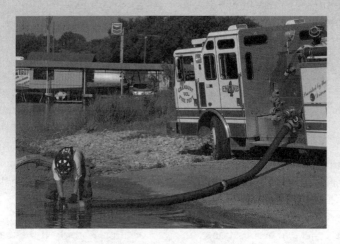

were all taken recently and during the light of day, Aaron could see that the homeowner had recently installed a 3-acre pond just 100 yards (91 m) downhill from the house. He knew from listening to the radio traffic that all water was currently being shuttled from hydrants more than 2 miles away. Aaron alerted Chief Andersen on the tactical channel, "Mountain Road Command, are you aware there is a large pond approximately 100 yards south of your location, and the gravel drive near the horse barn leads to it?"

Alerting is typically a direct communication and includes information that is meant to be immediately helpful to the team. Usually, the person alerting the team or the team leader has an understanding of the team goals and objectives, has situational awareness, and has information that needs to be shared immediately. As shown in the previous case, the person sharing the alert need not be physically present at the incident.

Challenge

A <u>challenge</u> is issued by a team member when he or she has already communicated a concern, either through probing questions or by issuing an alert. If the team or team leader does not acknowledge the probe or alert and begins the next phases of conflict resolution and discussion, the individual who recognizes an emergent problem may need to verbally challenge the situation and prepare to take the next step of emergency intervention. This is best done with a direct communication to the team leader, using the leader's name and rank (if appropriate) and clearly stating the following:

- What the observer sees or hears that he or she believes is a threat
- Why this appears to be a threat
- What the observer believes will occur if the threat is not immediately dealt with
- What the observer suggests the team leader do to counter the threat

Consider the following case. It takes place in an EMS setting, and because it involves a significant difference in hierarchy, it demonstrates a good method to properly phrase such a challenge.

CASE STUDY 6

Phil Orwalt was the captain in charge of Engine 16, and when his crew arrived at Skyline Boulevard and 232nd Avenue he could see the 2006 GMC Yukon had landed on its top in the deep ditch that ran parallel to Skyline. The 76-year-old male driver had been ejected and was laying to the rear of the vehicle, slightly downhill from the wreckage. Captain Orwalt took charge of the scene and was the designated Paramedic in Charge (or PIC).

Captain Orwalt had two members of his crew move to stabilize the patient while one pulled a hose line for protection. Shortly after his crew arrived at the

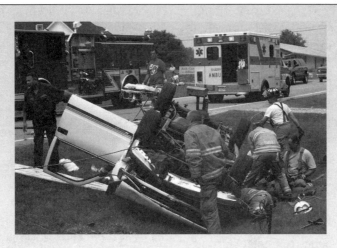

patient's side, Medic 401, the transport ambulance, arrived on scene. Riding along that evening was Dr. Turley, a well-known trauma surgeon from the local Level 1 trauma center. As Dr. Turley and the crew from Medic 401 entered the ditch, the patient went into cardiac arrest. CPR was started as further assessment was completed. Local protocols indicated that blunt trauma patients in cardiac arrest were declared dead at the scene if they had no vital signs and transport to the trauma center would take longer than 12 minutes. As the PIC, Captain Orwalt knew that the transport time would be in excess of 15 minutes, and this patient was dead.

At that moment, Captain Orwalt also smelled fuel leaking from the Yukon and decided to have his crew immediately move the patient from the ditch to an area of safety. At the same time, Dr. Turley had attached defibrillator pads from the Medic Unit's cardiac monitor and was preparing to give the patient a shock. Captain Orwalt first asked the doctor what his intentions were (sense making and probing). When he got no response, and with his understanding of the situation and the risks involved, Captain Orwalt alerted the doctor and medic crew to the potential danger of the procedure by stating, "There is a gas leak, defibrillation could cause a dangerous spark." His alert, although a direct statement, was not specifically directed at any one person. (His two fire fighters, however, immediately backed away from the patient and climbed out of the ditch.) Again, there was no response from the physician as he fiddled with the knobs and prepared to deliver the shock.

Captain Orwalt then stepped forward into the circle of medics, placed his hand on top of the cardiac monitor, and spoke directly to the trauma physician: "Dr. Turley, I understand you want to deliver a shock to this patient. However, I need to warn you that there is a gas leak from the vehicle that could ignite as soon as you push that button. I recommend we move the patient immediately to a safer position before you begin treatment."

This is a challenge, and it is more direct than an alert in that it may involve a team member physically placing him- or herself in the action circle, prepared to take the next step of emergency intervention.

Captain Orwalt said he resisted the urge to simply have his fire fighter open the hose line. He also elected not to engage the physician in discussing protocols related to resuscitation at that moment; that could wait until the team was in a safer position. The physician later pulled him aside and thanked him for the warning. During a postincident critique, the fire fighters discussed at length how these situations should be handled.

As Captain Orwalt told his crew, "Next time it might be me making the poor decision and you stepping in to ensure we don't collectively do something stupid."

Emergency Intervention

The most extreme step anyone can take in the advocacy phase of the CRM communication loop is **emergency intervention (EI)**. EI is when a team member takes a direct action to immediately save an individual or the team from harm. It is rare and usually indicates one of two situations: either a complete breakdown in communications within the team or an immediate critical threat where there is no time to engage in alerting or challenging.

If Dr. Turley had not responded to Captain Orwalt's challenge in the preceding example, Captain Orwalt may have elected to use one of several emergency interventions. He could have physically pulled the physician away from the monitor, but any time someone engages in behavior that involves physically touching, pushing, or pulling another person, he or she invites severe conflict and misunderstanding (which, it can be argued, is better than the alternative, which can be death). Another, less threatening move would have been to reach over and shut off the cardiac monitor or to pull off the pads and direct the crew to move the patient immediately.

During CRM training, it is vitally important to have team members engage in these types of practice scenarios to provide them with tools to use when they face real situations that are threatening to their team. This type of training also helps leaders pick up on cues that they may be missing from team members.

Conflict Resolution

Few people truly enjoy conflict, yet it is a necessary part of team dynamics and a by-product of bringing together any group of high-performance individuals with experience and strong opinions. Add the components of personal danger, time pressure, and a high-stakes outcome, and it is a recipe for poor performance. However, as mentioned earlier, it is not the absence of conflict that makes a good team, but the manner in which team members handle it. The key to **conflict resolution** revolves around the saying, "*what* is right, not *who* is right." (See **FIGURE 6.4**.) Conflict resolution is a range of processes aimed at alleviating or eliminating sources of conflict; these generally include negotiation, mediation, and diplomacy. It is important to remember that CRM is not team decision making. Most teams using CRM principles are not formed on democratic principles, but instead have a hierarchy related to rank and experience. Because teams have a designated leader and may also have domain experts who are informal leaders, it is critically important for team members to understand how they should handle conflict when it inevitably occurs.

First, leaders (formal or informal) carefully need to examine their own response and feelings when a team member probes or alerts. Typically, an initial response is the physical flush that comes with being embarrassed or challenged by someone else, particularly if a leader has yet to develop a personal relationship with the team member providing the challenge. By recognizing internal physical and emotional signals, team leaders can respond not with emotion but with curiosity and respect. All humans suffer from some cognitive dissonance when they face the prospect that they may have made a mistake, missed an important cue, or were otherwise found to be lacking. An initial human response is to reduce that feeling of discomfort, that dissonance, by either defending one's position (or decision) or attacking the sender of the message to minimize that person's standing.

A cardinal rule in conflict resolution—and one of the most difficult to employ—is for team members to stay focused on the mission or the issue at hand. Therefore, all participants must continually remind themselves to devote all attention to the current source of conflict. Conflict resolution is not the place to address past disputes. Biases need to be put aside. The primary goal is for everyone involved to concentrate all efforts on resolution.

Humans experience a biologic response to emotional challenges. A portion of the human brain called the amygdala controls immediate response to external

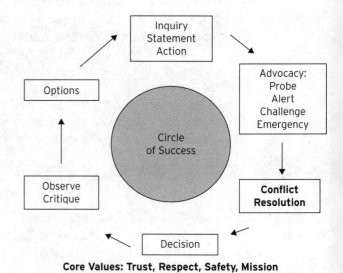

FIGURE 6.4 Conflict resolution focuses on determining what is right, rather than who is right.

stimuli. The amygdala evaluates incoming stimuli for any sign indicating trouble: "Is this something that could hurt or embarrass me? Is it something I fear?" If the answer is yes, then the amygdala can take control of a person's actions before his or her thinking brain, the neocortex, even has time to come to a decision.

It is helpful to think of *emotional response* as high-speed wireless connectivity and *reasoning* as dial-up. An immediate emotional reaction can be harsh, personally protective, and counterproductive. Most people do not recognize when they have reacted in an irrational manner. Once an individual becomes aware of the sensations and triggers, however, he or she can begin to practice more control when responding to conflict. Good leaders are self-aware enough to understand this phenomenon and have developed strategies for dealing with it. (See **FIGURE 6.5**.)

Behavioral health specialist Bill Hollis of Portland, Oregon focuses his professional efforts on teams that are composed of fire fighters, paramedics, police, and emergency dispatchers. His well-used advice for leaders and team members who find themselves reacting negatively to an external stimulus is "Be curious." Team leaders and members should be curious about why their body reacts the way it does during conflict, why the other person sees them the way he or she does, what the person has to say, and why he or she has a different perception of the same situation.

This type of curiosity is extraordinarily valuable. It allows people metaphorically to step back from the immediate situation and take stock of their own perceptions, feelings, and biases. It also allows people on one side of a conflict to place themselves directly in the other person's position to see whether they can understand the opposing perception and concerns.

When managing conflict at this stage in the CRM communication loop (it is important to remember that this loop often takes only seconds to complete in real-time situations), it is helpful to understand that complete resolution of the conflict is not likely to occur until after the situation is entirely concluded and more time can be spent discussing options. In the midst of any incident, the most anyone can hope for is to achieve an understanding of what the concerns are and why they exist. Sometimes the best that team leaders and decision makers can do, particularly if they are not planning on changing the strategy even after hearing the concern, is to communicate clearly to the individual expressing the concern that they understand what he or she is saying, recognize the potential impact on team operations, and value the input.

Decision

As indicated, the primary reason to employ CRM principles is to provide a collective situational awareness to the team or crew. Whether it is a physician, police sergeant, lead paramedic, company officer, or chief, there must be an identified leader in every team who can make decisions. (See **FIGURE 6.6**.) Teams without leaders tend to wander among options, with no one person assuming responsibility for the team's actions or the outcome, as the following scenario depicts.

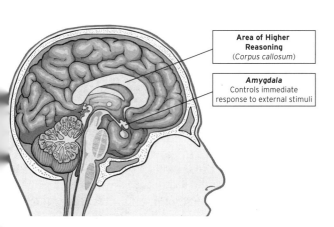

FIGURE 6.5 The amygdala controls our immediate response to external stimuli. Response time from the amygdala to higher reasoning is delayed approximately 30 seconds. A team leader must lead by example, to teach crew members to keep immediate emotional response in check when attempting to resolve conflict.

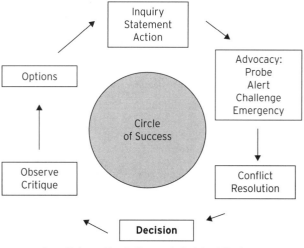

FIGURE 6.6 The team leader is responsible for guiding his or her crew toward making a decision about using a particular strategy during emergency response.

CASE STUDY 7

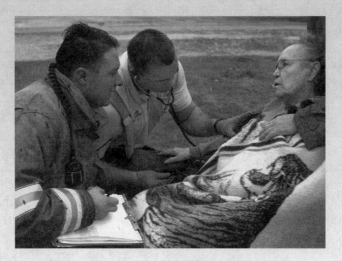

Paramedic Engine 35 and Medic 16, an ambulance, arrive simultaneously at the home of 85-year-old Greta Holmes, who has called 9-1-1 for mild shortness of breath and fainting. On this day, there are three paramedics among the four crew members on Engine 35: the officer, Mike Inverti; the apparatus operator, Jose Huerta; and Mary-Ann Jillian, one of the two fire fighters. The fourth fire fighter, Jim Knowlton, is an EMT-Basic with more than 18 years of experience. Additionally, Medic 16 is staffed with two paramedics.

Upon entering the home, the senior paramedic from Medic 16 begins questioning Greta, who appears to be in some distress. She is pale, with clammy skin, and she is slightly slow to respond to their questions. The other paramedic on the ambulance begins to place a cardiac monitor on the patient.

While this is taking place, Captain-Paramedic Mike Inverti steps out of the room to question the family and get the medical history. The AO-Paramedic Huerta completes a set of vital signs and reports a blood pressure of 130/96, pulse rate of 30, and a respiratory rate of 32. The cardiac monitor is now attached and shows the patient's bradycardia rhythm. Fire Fighter/Paramedic Jillian starts an intravenous line on Greta's left arm. All medics suddenly become fixated on the cardiac monitor's bradycardia, and a decision is made to administer the patient atropine 0.5 mg intravenously.

Fire Fighter/EMT Knowlton suggests to the paramedics present that atropine is not indicated, but receives no verbal response, and exits to find his officer. Meanwhile, the patient receives the medication.

Upon returning to the station, Captain-Paramedic Inverti followed up with the receiving hospital and confirmed that Greta was suffering from a stroke. She had a history of hypertension and anticoagulant therapy, and a recent history of a small cerebrovascular accident (CVA). Upon learning of the history, it became apparent to all that a medication error was made. With so many paramedics on the scene, there was a "diffusing of authority." This diffusion is a common failure of teams, particularly when there is a weak leader or the leader is not immediately present when the decision are being made.

Although the EMT-Basic, an 18-year veteran, commented on the need to reconsider the therapy being discussed in the room, his comments were disregarded by the paramedic holding the medication because the EMT Basic was seen as a person without paramedic training and therefore his opinion was less valuable.

When the medical director questioned the crew none of the paramedics recalled why atropine was draw up and administered. (See **FIGURE 6.7**.) One paramedic remembered a person saying, "It's a bradycardia on the monitor," while another recalled asking "Is it symptomatic?" and not receiving an answer; yet another recalls thinking to himself "What exactly qualifies as symptomatic?" The medic administering the drug recalled small bits of each of the other paramedics' comments. Importantly, no one expressed these concerns out loud, and no one took responsibility to step back and assume the lead role.

This was an experienced crew with excellent working relationships between personnel. Although many other factors could have complicated this situation, the predominant failure was one of leadership. A good team, after suffering such a failure, revisits the situation and discusses what might have been barriers to good communication. For example, were they fatigued? Was a team member not familiar with the crew and unwilling to speak up?

One of the duties of a good leader is to take responsibility for team performance. Good leaders are decisive, yet they are also empathetic and careful listeners. A decision should be made when team members get behind the group's efforts, even if one of them does not necessarily agree with the chosen course. During the next phase, such a team member needs to provide input because the entire team witnesses events unfold after a decision is made. Additionally, leaders must keep in mind that during critical communication events many decisions are made and the constant flow of communication is critical. If a leader and the team have reevaluated their strategy and decided to employ a new one, it is imperative that the entire team be aware of this, along with anyone else who may be affected. Decision making carries with it a great responsibility.

Observe and Critique

It can be said that if four fire fighters arrive at an extrication scene, then there are at least 16 different methods that could be employed to extricate the patient. Everyone thinks their idea is the best one, particularly if the idea isn't the one initially chosen.

After the decision to move forward with a particular strategy or tactic has been made, it is important for all team members to carefully observe the process and evaluate progress against the initially stated mission goals. (See **FIGURE 6.8**.) If something appears unsafe, if things aren't going according to plan, or if the individuals or equipment chosen for the task don't appear appropriate, a good team engages in critique conversation where they evaluate the operation on the fly. This should be constructive conversation and should include specifics: What isn't working as expected? Why might the problem exist? What can be done to modify the plan? These brief yet important communications lead to discussing options.

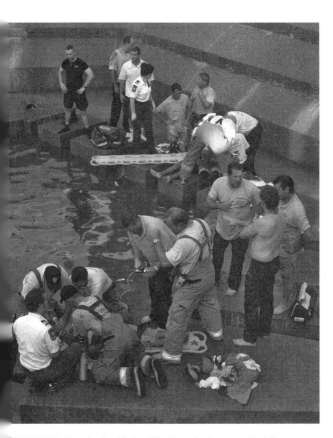

FIGURE 6.7 Clear leadership is critical in order to ensure that the proper medication is given to the patient.

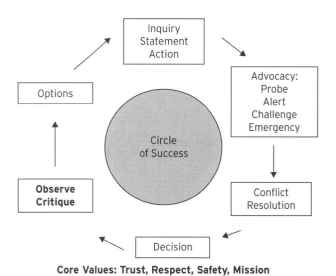

FIGURE 6.8 After a decision has been made, it is important for all team members to carefully evaluate an incident outcome against the initial mission goals.

In teaching CRM, it is important to identify *how* different members of a team observe and critique once a decision is made to take action. There are differences in what each team member will observe and consider important, depending on his or her level of experience and particular domain expertise. Observation leads to critique, and critique should be an open process because it brings out comments, statements, and questions that lead the team to discuss options, leading back to the inquiry phase. This is where good leaders shine: They encourage input, particularly when things start to get quiet. If team members are not commenting on their observations, they aren't collectively sharing their understanding of what they see.

For example, the following exchange took place on a hazardous materials incident at a large commercial building.

CASE STUDY 8

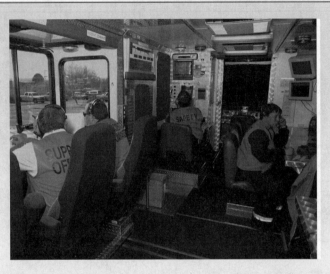

The incident commander had a multidisciplinary group of law enforcement, EMS, fire, hazardous materials, and public works experts within his unified command team. At one point, the team made a decision to prepare a specific medical antidote kit that could be readily available in the event any rescuer came into contact with the hazardous material.

As the medically trained members of the team gave directions on how to assemble the antidote kit, the hazardous materials expert observed the activity. Although he was acutely familiar with the hazards associated with the spilled chemical, he did not understand the pharmacology of how the antidote was being prepared. He had questions about the way the medical crew was handling the medications used in the antidote. He hesitated in asking questions, however, because he did not have any expertise in the medical aspect of preparing an antidote.

As the command team managed several activities, the incident commander noted that several members were quietly watching the medical experts. The commander simply asked the question, "Is everyone OK with what we're doing?" At that moment, the hazardous materials technician spoke up and said, "I'm no expert on how to use all these medications together, but is everyone aware that two of those medications contain chemicals that will spontaneously combust if they are put together without the third chemical?" According to the incident commander, the pause that followed allowed everyone to gain a shared understanding of the potential problems that could result if they continued. Needless to say, other options were discussed and implemented.

In teaching CRM, educators should carefully assess how actively each participating team member engages in observing and critiquing. They can evaluate this by watching how team members ask questions and by assessing team members' motivation and ability to clarify their understanding of how the situation is developing.

Discuss Options

As the team critiques their work and its results, they may decide that other options are necessary. (See **FIGURE 6.9**.) In critical situations that develop over a period of time, this duty is often relegated to a planning section. Within the small team environment and during rapidly developing situations, options are often presented as questions that are posed to the group. Options are a necessary part of emergency operations in any dynamic environment. Field operators in EMS, law enforcement, fire, and rescue services recognize that even though a team has determined a course of action, they must always evaluate other options. In this context, many team leaders start ordering resources and planning logistically to implement one of several alternatives.

Consider the following case.

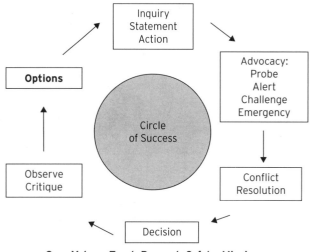

FIGURE 6.9 After a thorough assessment of their work, a team may decide that other tactical options need to be considered.

CASE STUDY 9

Urban Search and Rescue (USAR) Team 51 had been called to a new residential development to assist in extricating a worker who was pinned in a trench collapse. The rescue was complicated. The ground had been disturbed several times, making it very unstable. In addition, other excavation workers were highly agitated, angry that the fire department was working "too slowly" to pull out their friend and coworker. The rescue team had hundreds of hours in training for this type of event, but only one of the eight USAR members had actually ever responded to a real trench rescue. Their primary tactic included placing large reinforced panels into the trench and securing them with pneumatic shoring devices.

As USAR Fire Fighter Jones from Rescue 51 placed the next panel to stabilize the trench wall, he called out to USAR Fire Fighter Kline to fire the airshore and pin the fourth panel against the one on the opposite side of the open channel. They both could see that dirt was still freely running into the trench from one end, threatening to further bury their victim. Captain Ginther, in charge of the team, realized that the shoring operation would take more time than they had and the victim would likely not survive any more pressure from the moving earth. He openly called across the trench to the rest of his team, "What are our options, folks?"

Kline recognized that the large excavator nearby could be used to provide stabilization for the final two trench panels, and he knew how to run the machine. However, he also knew that the vibration from starting and moving it could further exacerbate the problem and cause more dirt to fall on the

(continues)

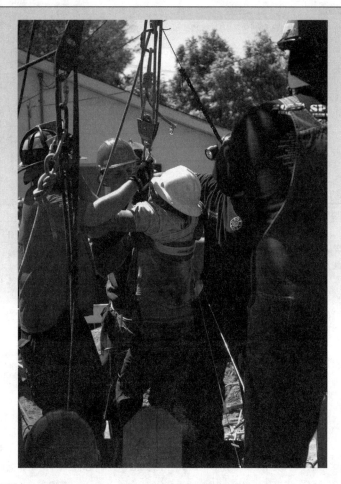

victim. Kline called out and discussed his option: "I can move the excavator 10 feet to the left and place both of the final panels at once. The risks are that the panels could be difficult to control as they enter the trench, but we can tie them off and guide them, and that the excavator may vibrate dirt onto the victim."

Discussing options moves the team back into the beginning phase of the CRM loop: They had a plan, they made a decision on what to do, they evaluated their evolving circumstances, and they proposed options and outlined risk. The new option returns to the beginning of the process and is considered an inquiry ("What do you think of Plan B?"), and team members can openly agree with the idea or probe further to develop any concerns.

In this case, the team from Rescue 51 chose to go with Plan B, and although they had several moments where operations were stopped so that they could further critique their actions, the victim was successfully extricated from the trench without any injuries to the rescue crew.

Summary

Using a step-by-step model to outline the critical phases in team communication helps team members recognize how and when they should participate in gaining a collective understanding of the situation, plus the risks and benefits associated with each decision.

By emphasizing that *inquiry* is simply an opening for communication and that it can be represented in many different forms (a question, statement, order, behavior, or action), individuals can see that every mode of communication is an opening for further clarification and understanding.

The process of advocacy is either active or passive. Every member of a team must recognize that there are two methods of stating approval in a team environment (a person states their approval or says nothing) and only one method for clearly articulating a difference of opinion (respectfully providing feedback on why he or she thinks the proposed action or behavior won't be effective or safe).

Once team members have respectfully provided input, the process of conflict resolution takes place. This is an exercise in curiosity in which every team member develops a genuine curiosity regarding any differences of opinion. If a conflict in opinion cannot be resolved, the team at least arrives at a shared understanding of the potential outcomes.

The leader, who takes responsibility for any failure and encourages the team to provide immediate feedback, typically makes decisions.

Active observation and open critique are critical components for success. Everyone has a slightly different viewpoint, and all team members focus on slightly different perspectives as the event unfolds. Good team leaders actively encourage their team members to give feedback while they actively observe the results of decisions.

Discussing options leaves open the opportunities that exist in a dynamic working environment. This phase allows further inquiry to develop, and this thinking out loud can be a helpful way for team members to clarify their current understanding of the situation and also provide input on potential resolutions.

In training for CRM, **experiential learning** is critical. Experiential learning is the process of making meaning from direct experience. Setting course objectives that are associated with individual and team competence, motivation, ability, and knowledge is important. Skill in CRM is primarily associated with team members understanding their own behavior as individuals, how they interact with team members, and how they cognitively process information that is presented in a rapid and dynamic way.

Wrap Up

Ready for Review

- Effective CRM encompasses a range of competencies, skills, and behaviors, including situational awareness, problem solving, decision making, teamwork, leadership, followership, and self-awareness. These cognitive and interpersonal capabilities must be developed and practiced like any technical skill. Team members also must have technical proficiency in certain areas, such as starting an IV, operating a hose line, doing a surgical procedure, and tying a knot.
- The primary reason to employ CRM principles is to provide a collective situational awareness to the team or crew.
- The CRM model contains several key elements, all of them integral to gaining a shared understanding within a culture of learning and mutual respect. These elements are inquiry, advocacy, conflict resolution, decision, observe and critique, and discuss options.
- Questioning authority, either hierarchical or expert, is a daunting task. There are two methods team members can use to state approval in a team environment: state approval or say nothing. There is only one method for team members to clearly articulate a difference of opinion: to respectfully provide feedback on why the proposed action or behavior won't be effective or safe.
- An inquiry is simply an opening for communication that can be presented in many different forms: as a question, statement, order, behavior, or action. Perceiving inquiries in this way allows individuals to see that every mode of communication is an opening for further clarification and understanding.

Vital Vocabulary

Alert When a team member simply and clearly states what he or she is seeing or experiencing that might compromise the mission or objective.

Challenge More direct than an alert; when a team member physically moves into the action circle, prepared to take the next step of emergency intervention.

Coherence When truth aligns with some specified set of sentences, propositions, or beliefs.

Conflict resolution A range of processes aimed at alleviating or eliminating sources of conflict; generally includes negotiation, mediation, and diplomacy.

Emergency intervention (EI) When a team member takes a direct action to immediately save an individual or the team from harm.

Experiential learning The process of making meaning from direct experience.

Recognition-primed decision making When a responder *recognizes* a situation based on his or her experience and is *primed* to act in a certain way based on previous successful (or unsuccessful) outcome.

Sense making The ability or attempt to make sense of an ambiguous situation.

Assessment in Action

1. The primary reason to employ CRM principles is:
   A. for quality assurance purposes.
   B. to create team decision making.
   C. to allow fairness to all team members.
   D. to provide a collective situational awareness to the team or crew.
2. An emergency intervention is:
   A. a disciplinary process.
   B. required often at incidents.
   C. the highest level of advocacy in the circle of success.
   D. required of Advanced Life Support (ALS) trained personnel.
3. Sense making:
   A. occurs when a team member is unable to reconcile an ambiguous situation.
   B. is a group activity.
   C. should be discouraged.
   D. requires special training.
4. Coherence in communication deals with:
   A. establishing protocols.
   B. written orders.
   C. nonemergent situations.
   D. how well the receiver understands the message.

In-Classroom Activity

1. Apply the circle of success to the two opening scenarios in this chapter.
2. Role-play a part in the following scenarios using the PACE procedure:
   - Recognizing a bad anchor on a technical rescue involving high-angle extraction
   - Identifying a live fire exercise that is not National Fire Protection Association (NFPA) compliant
   - A decision by an aeromedical crew to take a flight when bad weather approaches
   - A decision to cancel a helicopter en route to a traumatic cardiac arrest
   - A decision to force entry into a building with an automated alarm

References

1. Bill Hollis, "Curiosity and Conflict." (Portland, OR: self-published material, 2008).
2. Robert O. Besco, "To Intervene or Not to Intervene? The Co-Pilot's Catch 22" (white paper, 2004), http://www.crm-devel.org/resources/paper/PACE.PDF.

7

Leaders, Followers, and Teamwork

Objectives

- Describe how leaders envision goals and set clear objectives.
- Describe how the behaviors of delegating authority, taking responsibility, and gaining commitment create a small, high-performance team.
- Describe the leader's ability to maintain a dynamic situational assessment.
- Describe how to understand individual and team limitations.
- Describe the leader's ability to adjust.
- Describe how to value team diversity.
- Describe how to listen aggressively and with curiosity.
- Describe the role of the mentor in leadership.
- Describe how to manage relationships as a leader.
- Define an effective follower.
- Define the behaviors that are hazardous to team cohesion.

CASE STUDY 1

At approximately 15:45 PM, Strike Team 2642 carefully navigated the one-lane gravel road that led to Rodgers Ridge, where they had been ordered to engage in some brush clearing and structural defense operations around three large vacation homes that were distributed across the ridge top. Captain Doug Chandler was leading a strike team for the first time, and he cautiously watched the two separate smoke columns that spouted from the 1600-acre Camp Creek Fire and the 2300-acre Jones Ranch Fire in the valley just beyond the ridge. For the moment, the wind was at their backs and would be pushing the fire away from the ridge.

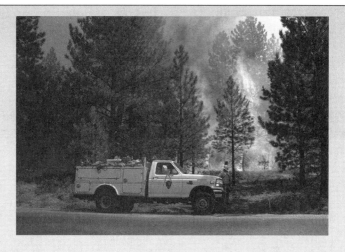

The five units that made up Captain Chandler's strike team were all heavy brush (HB) units, each staffed with one officer and three fire fighters and carrying 500 gallons (1892.5 liters) of water, foam, and the normal complement of tools. As they reached the large turnaround near the ridge top, the captain noted that all three homes were built within 50 ft (15.2 m) of each other, with one being the closest to the lip of the canyon, and the other two set back along a single driveway that led off the main road. At 4:20 PM, Captain Chandler ordered two of his brush units, HB26 and HB27, to proceed all the way down the driveway to the house at the end and to "prepare the residence house for defensive operations." He sent brush units HB28 and HB29 to the two remaining houses and ordered them to prep those structures, while he stayed in a "lookout" position in HB25 near the driveway entrance.

At 4:27 PM, Captain Chandler received a call on his cell phone from the Operations Division. They informed him that the weather was due to change, and that he could expect temperatures to increase for another 30 minutes to a high of 94°F. Humidity was expected to stay extremely low, and the winds were to turn 180° by 7:00 PM. Captain Chandler in turn contacted his strike team by radio, telling them, "Strike Team 2642, all units, just be advised we're due for a wind change." He issued no further orders, and radio records showed that only HB26 acknowledged the message. Eighteen minutes later, at 4:45 PM, Captain Chandler in HB25 again communicated a message to his strike team: "ST 2642, all units, from my position it appears the wind has changed and may be pushing the fire toward the ridge." This time, both HB26 and HB27 acknowledged, both with the single word "Copy."

Just 12 minutes later, at 4:57 PM, HB26 frantically radioed that they were in danger. "HB26 and 27 here, we've ... we've got lots of fire rolling toward us and it appears it'll cut between our location and yours." (Postincident analysis indicated the fire was moving at a speed of greater than 10 ft per second [3.1 m per second] at that point.)

As Captain Chandler attempted to radio his Operations Division for assistance, he was "walked on" by HB26, who again called out, "27 from 26 ... we're taking cover inside the house, you should follow us."

At this point, Captain Chandler ordered HB28 and HB29 to "pull back immediately from your positions, pull back to the gravel turnaround where my rig is based." He then radioed, "Break ... HB26, what do you need?" HB26 responded, "The fire has rolled over our position ... both units HB26 and HB27 are on fire. We are in the house in need of assistance."

Remarkably, no personnel were seriously injured in this event. However, two brush units were lost and eight fire fighters nearly lost their lives. A postincident analysis would place significant weight on the lack of leadership exhibited not only by Captain Chandler, but by the junior officers who staffed each brush unit. At no point did Chandler clarify the objectives, and neither did he discuss alternative plans about what crews should do if the fire approached. In addition, when the wind changed direction, at least 10 minutes passed in which the fire fighters could have pulled out and headed for a safety zone.

Books and studies on leadership and those attributes necessary to be a good leader are numerous. Certainly, some individuals seem to just have what it takes to be a good leader. However, specific behaviors seem to stand out when it comes to small team leadership. (See **FIGURE 7.1**.) These behaviors are often categorized as knowledge, skills, and attitudes (KSAs) and include the following:

- Envisioning goals and setting clear objectives
- Delegating authority; taking responsibility
- Gaining commitment and motivating
- Maintaining a dynamic situational assessment
- Understanding individual and team limitations
- Ability to adjust
- Valuing team diversity
- Ability to listen aggressively and with curiosity
- Setting clear expectations

Additionally, leaders can and should be good mentors. Mentoring someone takes work, and it demonstrates an unselfish understanding of what the team and the organization need to survive and thrive.

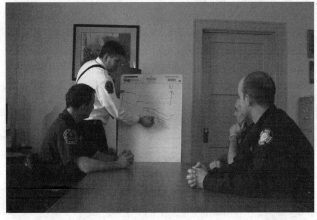

FIGURE 7.1 Specific behaviors seem to stand out when it comes to small team leadership.

Leaders: Envisioning Goals and Setting Clear Objectives

Most teams are created for a specific purpose—to get something done. Whether that is performing surgery on a patient, putting out a fire, capturing a dangerous criminal, caring for a cardiac arrest victim, or helping a city recover from a disaster, teams come together to accomplish a common set of objectives.

The team leader typically needs to consider the number and type of objectives, their clarity, and their priority, with input from team members. Because often there are competing objectives and multiple methods for achieving them, effective leaders communicate what they perceive to be the priorities and then ask for input. They set a direction for the team. This ability requires the following skills:

1. Leaders must be able to get the team's attention and hold it while distractions occur.

Gaining and holding the team's attention can be done using hierarchy (the leader's authority position), but a leader usually has more success by employing subtle people skills. For example, some leaders have been very successful in getting and holding the team's attention by using steady eye contact and a quiet, calm tone of voice that requires the team members to listen actively. This method also can help reduce the tension level.

2. Leaders must be able to gain situational awareness, identify goals, and set specific and achievable objectives.

Strong leaders understand that goals can be identified only after they have a sense of what is happening and what needs to be done. As discussed earlier, situational awareness in a team environment requires activating a feedback loop: asking for input, requesting updates, and checking in with each individual. An important point to remember is that leaders should expect to receive unpleasant information if they openly ask for input. The news they receive may not be what they anticipate, yet it is critical that leaders maintain a sense of active curiosity, particularly if they perceive something differently from how a reporting team member perceives it.

3. Leaders must have the ability to ensure that all team members understand the team's stated goals and objectives.

Misunderstandings are common in team communication. Good leaders desire a shared understanding among team members where goals and objectives have a common definition. Leaders can achieve shared understanding by asking team members to restate the specific goal or objective. Questions such as "What do you think we need to do now?" or "What did you hear me ask for?" help provide clarification, particularly if the goal includes multiple steps or requires the involvement of other teams for a successful outcome.

Delegating Authority, Taking Responsibility, and Gaining Commitment

The behaviors of delegating authority, taking responsibility, and gaining commitment are related, particularly in the context of the small, high-performance team.

Delegating Authority

If leaders do not delegate authority, it is unlikely they will gain commitment from team members. Delegating authority sounds like an easy task, and many leaders claim they do it regularly. However, true delegation is when a leader gives an individual who has been assigned a task both the authority and responsibility to accomplish that task. To delegate successfully, leaders should be sure to do the following:

1. Clearly state the end result that is desired. Ask the individual to repeat what he or she sees as the goal. Leaders must ensure that this vision is congruent with their own.
2. Give the delegate the resources he or she needs to accomplish the task safely and in the time frame specified.
3. Determine whether the individual delegated the task will need guidance. A delicate balance must be maintained between providing guidance and dictating the task. If the leader steps in to manage or dictate the process, the individual may not learn (or may become resentful). In addition, if the leader dictates a specific process that must be followed, little innovation will occur. This is like the difference between giving someone a road map with specific step-by-step directions and giving the person a compass, where the individual understands the direction to go and the goal, but is left to his or her own skill and experience to get there.

When leaders delegate authority, they must accept the risk that the mission objectives may not be carried out exactly like they had envisioned and that novice team members may take extra time or make mistakes. An applicable adage is "don't let the perfect be the enemy of the good." Leaders may have a clear picture in mind of how the perfect mission should be carried out or how a specific objective should be accomplished but must realize that team members learn by working through the challenges they face. This doesn't mean that leaders let team members spiral down and fail. Leaders must watch closely, offer advice when necessary, coach regularly, and give team members a compass rather than a road map to find their way through problems.

Taking Responsibility

Regardless of how well teams plan and execute strategy during dynamic events, such as structure fires, emergency medical incidents, or critical care scenarios, there are times when mistakes occur. As noted in Chapter 3, mistakes are opportunities for leaders to learn about their team, abilities, and the limits of their knowledge. If a mistake occurs, the leader should assume responsibility for the error, own it as a team failure, and ensure that the team learns from it by engaging in thorough debriefing. Any efforts to point fingers and assign blame fracture teams. Additionally, team members will be reluctant to take on new challenges if they think the consequence of error is a personal reckoning.

CASE STUDY 2

As a new paramedic, Paul LeSage had a good leader to follow. Larry set a good example, was a continual learner, and delegated tasks to Paul on a regular basis. Larry demonstrated that he trusted Paul, and when he fell down, Larry was always there to pick him up and discuss what could have been done differently. He really became a leader to Paul. But Paul was but a month into his new career when his unit responded to a cardiac arrest. Back in those days, before defibrillating a patient, a connective gel paste had to be applied to the paddles of the defibrillator and the paddles had to be rubbed together before placing them on the patient's chest. In the medical kits, the tube of cardiac gel was kept in the bottom, very close to another tube that looked nearly identical. The second tube held glucose paste, an extremely

(continues)

> sticky substance that was squeezed into the mouths of conscious diabetics to increase their blood glucose level. Paul's partner and leader, Larry, told him to defibrillate the patient as other seasoned medics started IVs, secured the airway, and prepared medications.
>
> Paul reached into the bottom of the kit and grabbed a tube, generously squeezing a large dollop of gel onto the paddles. Paul then slapped them together with the intent of rubbing them and spreading the gel around. However, the paddles immediately stuck together as if with glue; it was nearly impossible to separate them. When Paul finally pulled them apart, long gooey strings of glucose dripped off the face of the paddles. Larry quickly took the paddles from Paul, placed them on the patient's chest, yelled "Clear!" and delivered a shock to the man. As a strong smell of burned sugar wafted up, Larry looked at the other medics, stated, "My fault, I left the tubes together this morning at inventory," and continued the resuscitation. Of course, it wasn't his fault; Paul should have looked more closely at the tubes before applying the gel.
>
> Paul learned several valuable lessons that day. One, obviously, was to double-check everything. More important, Paul learned that teamwork includes delegating tasks, and it also means sharing responsibility, particularly for the leader. Last, Paul learned that a sense of humor can carry a person through nearly anything and can defuse a situation if used properly. Needless to say, after that Paul would've followed Larry anywhere. Paul felt an obligation and therefore was committed to his success.

Gaining Commitment

How does a leader gain commitment, and why is it important? When looking up the word *commitment*, *obligation* and *dedication* are key descriptive words in the definition. Followers who feel an obligation to team success and who are dedicated to the relationship function at a high level. Committed followers work at a high level of performance because no one individual wants to let the team down. Commitment among team members gives a leader a powerful tool: a collective of individuals who believe in the goals, believe in themselves, and importantly, look out for each other and help each other when one fails.

The Leader's Ability to Maintain a Dynamic Situational Assessment

There is an old, popular t-shirt one can find at many different collectible shops. On the t-shirt is printed the following words: "I am their leader.... Which way did they go?" Leaders, obviously, need to be aware of what's happening if they are to respond in an appropriate manner. They need to know what their team sees, which way they are going, and what the risks are. It is impossible for leaders to set goals and objectives if they do not understand the situation. Leaders need not be able to perceive the outcome, but they should have enough understanding of how a situation is unfolding to be able to engage their team constructively and safely. Good followers, on the other hand, help the leader by providing inputs that allow for a dynamic situational assessment. Dynamic situational assessment is conducted by soliciting continual feedback from all relevant input sources, particularly other team members and those involved in front-line operations. It's important for a leader to ask questions, clarify, and restate to minimize misunderstanding and to diversify their sources of information to gain insight.

As discussed earlier, one person's input can be another's distraction. So, it is important for leaders to clarify for other team members what sources they believe are necessary for the dynamic, ongoing situational assessment. It is equally important for followers to speak up if they need additional resources to keep up their own situational awareness. Additionally, if a leader shuts down a perceived source of distraction (e.g., a radio channel or a live news feed), it is essential for followers to immediately inform the leader if they need that particular information source.

Understanding Individual and Team Limitations

No one likes to be embarrassed or to look incompetent in front of others. Effective leaders do their best to understand the limits of each team member's experience and training prior to engaging in a critical operation. Although this isn't always possible—sometimes teams are put together immediately prior to a mission—it is surprising how many times teams have worked together for days, weeks, and even months without anyone on the team truly understanding the degree of experience and talent that each member possesses.

Good leaders ask questions early in their team's deployment. In some cases, this questioning can take place in front of other team members (particularly if team members know each other and are comfortable with one another). In other situations, it can be better for a leader to ask some questions in private. Private questioning may not be possible, in which case it is important for the leader to maintain a neutral and curious tone to avoid offending team members. Questions such as, "How comfortable are you with that piece of equipment?" "What types of incidents have you responded to in the past?" "What jobs do you feel comfortable with?" "What types of situations make you uncomfortable?" help a leader define the limits of his team members' experience and skill sets.

It is equally important that team leaders apprise team members of their own experience, strengths, and weaknesses. Because a leader's strengths are usually also his or her greatest weaknesses, the leader should point out how a specific characteristic, such as assertiveness, for example, can also be a weakness in certain situations.

For example, one of the strengths of a leader who is task oriented is the ability to prioritize multiple issues and get them done quickly and efficiently. However, in the rush to get things prioritized and accomplished, the leader may miss some of the human dynamics in the environment. Perhaps a team member does not appreciate the process or has something going on in his personal or professional life that affects his performance. Therefore, the leader's strength is her ability to expeditiously and efficiently get things done, but her weakness is that such efficiency and speed tends to close out the collaborative, creative process of a team.

Leaders' limitations, then, are the blind spots that follow them around as they operate in "normal" mode. Their strength comes from an ability to understand their own nature and to openly ask the team (or more likely, a trusted individual team member) to watch out for this behavior and for signs that the leader's weakness is obstructing team performance.

Once a team is engaged and under time pressure, it is usually too late to determine how talented the members are with specific types of equipment or how much experience they have in particular domains. If the team fails because a leader assigned a task to someone who doesn't have the necessary training, experience, or cognitive ability to succeed, both the team member and the leader can find themselves in a risky situation, as the following account illustrates.

CASE STUDY 3

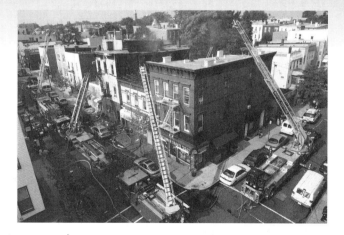

Lieutenant J.P. was known as "Dr. Disaster" because all the truly bad incidents seemed to occur on his shift. On this night, a very warm September evening,

(continues)

> J.P. and his crew of four fire fighters from TeleSquirt 51 and Rescue 51 were the third set of companies to arrive at a two-alarm apartment fire. The BellAir Apartments staggered down a hillside, so each adjoining apartment was between 4 and 6 ft (1.2 and 1.8 m) below its neighbor. On their arrival, J.P. could see from the front officer's seat that three units in the middle of the hill were fully involved.
>
> The crews from Station 51 were ordered to perform a quick primary search in the apartment that was immediately uphill from the series of involved units. The apartment to be searched and one of the units on fire shared a common wall. J.P. was also ordered to see whether he could confirm if there was fire involvement in the attic above the burning unit from his team's position in the uninvolved apartment.
>
> J.P. was a veteran, but among his five crew members one was a probationary fire fighter with less than 6 months of experience, and another had less than 2 years on the job. J.P.'s team entered the unit and began searching in near-zero visibility conditions (this was in the days before thermal imaging). Within a short time, they reported that the primary search was completed. At this point, J.P. asked his fire fighters to cut an "inspection hole" in the living room wall that, based on the construction features, he estimated would allow them to see into the attic of the adjoining unit. Because J.P. couldn't see the work being done but could hear the chainsaw running, he assumed everything was going according to plan. Soon, he would have an inspection hole that would allow him to view the adjoining attic space.
>
> However, the moment the chainsaw stopped, the temperature in the room immediately soared. Both fire fighters who had been cutting the inspection hole crawled over to J.P. and told him that heavy fire was "blowing through the hole" they had cut. J.P. told his crew to evacuate, made sure everyone was accounted for, and slid toward the wall to see if he could report the conditions to Incident Command. What he saw surprised him—the inspection hole was the size of a large window! After exiting the apartment, his crew initiated fire attack on the now-involved unit, quickly beating back the fire.

After the fact, J.P.'s probationary fire fighter told him that he had never been trained to cut an inspection hole. He had thought he needed to be able to stick his upper body through it to properly inspect whatever was on the other side.

The Ability to Adjust

Leaders help followers define what is important. Leaders also provide followers with specific guidance on just how much risk can be assumed in a given situation. In any dynamic incident, the risk profile can change often: What appeared safe moments ago may now be dangerous.

A common metaphor used to describe the ability to adjust is to imagine a leader pounding a stake in the ground. That stake is where the team makes its stand. Most times, the team hopes the leader places the stake after making a reasoned situational assessment. The leader conducts a personal risk analysis, checks the team, and uses his knowledge, skills, and experience to determine the limits of what can be done. However, even after the most comprehensive of assessments, things can change dramatically. This is where the dynamic situational assessment kicks in. Does the leader adjust? Or does he continue to make a stand? This is one of the most difficult situations for leaders, particularly new leaders, because moving their stake is a tacit admission that the first situational assessment was incomplete. Smart leaders understand that their responsibility is the safe functioning of their team. Their reputation does not hinge on whether they drove their stake in the ground in the wrong spot.

Unfortunately, there are many cases where blind ambition, stubbornness, or ego has intervened, and leaders are unable to adjust. They continue with their plan, continue to rally around their stake in the ground, regardless of the changing situation. This is often when followers desert their leaders for their own safety and for the safety of their team. Consider the following case.

CASE STUDY 4

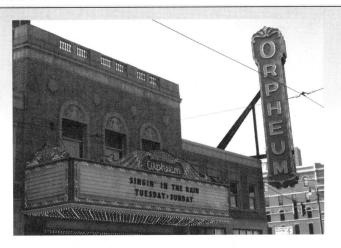

Battalion Chief Gregory worked for a large metropolitan fire department and was known to be a cranky, cantankerous guy. When Captain Albert was a new fire fighter and had met the chief, Gregory had told the recruits that he'd been a fire chief "longer than you've been alive." Now that Captain Albert had 12 years of experience, he knew the chief to be a guy who had lots of experiences, but little "collective experience." In other words, he didn't seem interested in learning from his past experiences or the experiences of others.

The night of the Orpheum Theater incident, BC Gregory was in charge of five stations. Captain Albert, who normally worked at a fire station outside the core area in an older neighborhood, was working a call shift at Ladder 91, which was situated in the older part of downtown just four blocks from the theater. At 2:03 AM, Box Alarm 2122 was struck for a reported fire on the back loading dock of the Prism Meat Company, which shared an alley with the Orpheum Theater. Ladder 91 was the first to arrive, and once Captain Albert saw the volume of fire he ordered his apparatus operator to park at the corner of the theater building, which would give Engine 91 access to the alley and would also preposition the ladder in the event they had to make a defensive attack. Engine 91 grabbed a hydrant on the nearby corner, and the crew stretched hose lines down the alley to fight the fire. However, the lieutenant on Engine 91 quickly reported that even their 2½" (64-mm) hose line wasn't making a dent in the fire, and fire had moved from the Prism loading dock into the back wall and overhanging roof of the Orpheum Theater.

As additional units started to arrive, BC Gregory took command and ordered an interior attack from the front of the theater. Captain Albert, who was at the rear and had a good view of the amount of fire, suggested to BC Gregory that they order additional units. "Command from Ladder 91, we have

(continues)

> ... there is heavy involvement in the roof, it has entered the rear upper stage area, we'll probably want a second alarm."
>
> In recordings pulled from the incident, BC Gregory's response was as follows: "Thanks for the suggestion, Cap. We're downtown now, I think we can take this with one alarm." Shortly after Gregory's transmission, the rear wall of the Orpheum collapsed, critically injuring two fire fighters from Engine 91 and pushing heavy fire into the seating area and lobby, causing interior crews to withdraw. Ladder 91 was ordered to rescue Engine 91's crew, and still Chief Gregory did not call for more resources.

The postincident analysis, conducted by a firm hired to do the investigation, stated, "The unwillingness of the Incident Commander to allow others on scene to contribute to his overall situational awareness contributed to the poor outcome. In addition, Chief Gregory used terminology that appears to be condescending, and his failure to adjust to the changing conditions is indicative of a lack of leadership."

Good leaders are expected to evaluate risk continually, which means they need to be ready to make adjustments at a moment's notice and listen carefully for indications that the current strategy may not be working.

Valuing Team Diversity

One very specific reason for some of the errors made by veterans and experts in teams is their belief that if they aren't aware of something it is not happening. Experienced persons tend to overestimate their ability to know about everything that is taking place, missing potential blind spots. Recall that within the recognition-primed decision-making environment, experts and veterans choose a single course of action and modify as they go based on what they have learned from past practice. What they generally do not do is pay attention to the relevant written policies and procedures for similar situations. Experts and veterans are subject to missing cues that novice and non-expert members of the team may pick up, cues that are embedded in the rules and policies. The diversity in experience of team members must be considered.

In addition to diversity among levels of experience, diversity is associated with technical expertise, communication skills, physiology, and myriad other topics among a well-developed team. Leaders understand that occasionally one team member will shine because his or her particular skill set or domain expertise lent itself to that situation, in that context, at that time. Effective leaders ensure that everyone is given credit for the success of the team and encourage everyone to learn from their experiences.

By championing the diversity of team members and understanding domain experts' blind spots, leaders can enrich team experience and ensure better outcomes.

Listening Aggressively and with Curiosity

To listen aggressively does not mean to lean in and invade the space of the person speaking. Instead, it means to listen with a goal of truly understanding what the person is saying as well as what he or she means. This is most effectively done when the listener briefly restates what he or she thinks the intent is behind the communication and clarifies any time he or she does not fully understand.

The CRM loop emphasizes the risks associated with *asymmetrical coherence*, or what happens when one person speaks and another interprets the communication incorrectly. Leaders demonstrate effective behavior to their team when they clarify, probe, and actively engage in communication with the goal of reaching a shared understanding. Consider the following case.

> ### CASE STUDY 5
>
> Critical Care Flight Nurse Sue Galeski was in charge of running the resuscitation. She was very good at her job, and her flight paramedic enjoyed working with her. On this particular Friday afternoon, their medical helicopter had responded to Highway 18 near the town of Sheridan, a heavily traveled

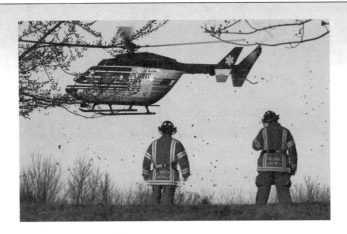

two-lane road that stretched between the Portland metro area and some central Oregon coastal communities. The flight crew and local paramedics worked diligently to try and save the life of a 36-year-old woman who had been thrown from her vehicle in a rollover accident.

As Sue prepped the patient for flight, she noted that the endotracheal tube that was being used to protect the airway appeared to be bent out of shape. She stated, "We need to take care of that kinked airway."

As the medics continued with their work, starting IVs, preparing additional paralytic medications, stabilizing the patient on a backboard, and bandaging an actively bleeding wound, Sue noticed that one of them was pulling out a King Airway, a secondary device that, at the time, was used when endotracheal intubation failed. In addition, she noticed another medic taking tape off the endotracheal tube, as if preparing to remove it.

Sue immediately spoke up and asked, "What did you hear me say?" One of the medics responded, "You said to take care of her with a King Airway, so that's what we're getting ready to do." In reliving the moment later, Sue said she wondered what could have been said to make them think she wanted them to pull out a perfectly good airway tube. Then, she suddenly realized that "kinked airway" sounded just like "King Airway."

The medics had simply been following orders—to use a King Airway. Sue was the expert, the leader, and she did a great job maintaining her situational awareness, probing, and correcting as needed.

Miscommunication has injured and killed many emergency providers. It will continue to be a major cause of incident failures, mistakes, and tragic outcomes. The effects can be minimized if individuals practice aggressive listening techniques and maintain a healthy curiosity when they see things that don't appear to mesh with their understanding of a situation.

Mentoring

Mentoring is very different from training, coaching, or assigning someone to a position of authority. A **mentor** is an individual, often older, who is more experienced in the domain and helps guide another individual's professional and personal development.

Dealing with complex issues and keeping an organization operating in a high-reliability mode requires guidance. As stated earlier, mentoring also demonstrates an unselfish approach in that a true mentor concedes some of her own power, through knowledge and delegation, to the person being mentored. This doesn't just help the individual who is being mentored grow—it also helps the organization by developing a deeper team. Any organization that works to expand its "bench strength" will be healthier when hard times hit or when someone unexpectedly drops out of the executive or leadership ranks.

In evaluating mentorship, it is often helpful for team members to ask themselves whether the guidance they seek (if looking for a mentor) or the guidance they are willing to provide (as a mentor) is for personal gain. True mentoring, whether given or received, is something that adds value to the organization, and personal or professional gain comes as a secondary benefit. When viewed in this context, others are more willing to provide critical input, and their own careers can be enriched by the mentoring experience. This behavior is critical for team success because the future leader will begin to develop a pattern of acting with the team's best interest first and an understanding that as the team succeeds so does the leader.

Consideration of the following points can contribute to successful mentoring:

- Write down in descriptive terms specific areas where you need assistance. Whether leading, managing projects, communicating in front of groups, or learning incident mitigation techniques, it is valuable to have clear objectives in mind when starting out.
- Describe what you would like from a mentor. Think hard about how others have been mentors to you in the past. What worked? What didn't?
- For each area in which you desire assistance, think about someone you respect in that particular domain and consider whether they will listen to you. Will you also be willing to listen to that individual? How can his mentoring of you bring that person benefit as well?
- Present your request to your future mentor with enough context for the person to understand your objective, your needs, and your concerns. Give her the approximate time commitment and tell her specifically why you asked her to mentor you. Be open to discussing with your future mentor how this relationship will affect you both. Don't be pushy or make the mentor feel guilty if she expresses concern. You want your mentor to be excited and pleased to be working with you.
- Consider ahead of time what benefits you can offer to your mentor. Are there things you can do for him? Be appreciative, discuss issues over a meal that you buy, offer some of your own insight, and think of ways you can honor his service to you and the organization. Never overload, abuse, or speak poorly of someone who is mentoring you, regardless of how your relationship ends, or you won't find another.

Remember that mentoring and leading require sharing knowledge. Many people think that knowledge is power, and they are reluctant to share their knowledge because they fear losing control or relevance. However, the more knowledge mentors give away, the more they accumulate, and the more relevant and powerful they become. This is why it is important for team leaders to support mentoring among the team and foster the types of relationships that make it easy for individuals to seek the assistance and wisdom they need.

Relationship Management for Leaders

"Managing relationships" sounds a bit technical and cold. However, relationship management is a crucial skill that includes diplomacy and the ability to find common ground. Diplomacy is about how a leader resolves his or her own personal conflicts and manages his or her feelings when confronted. Although CRM offers avenues to resolve team conflict, the very nature of the communication model ensures that some conflict will occur. It is helpful to remember that it is not the absence of conflict that makes a good team, but that good teams understand how to resolve conflict and manage side effects such as the feelings of low self-esteem that can result from being involved in conflict.

Within successful teams, leaders do not allow conflict to escalate to personal attacks or unresolved grudges. Tips for resolving specific team conflicts are outlined in the section titled "Conflict Resolution" in Chapter 6.

Effective relationship management starts with leaders' understanding of their own emotional intelligence. Every team leader can remember an instance (or two) when they made a comment during an incident or during an interpersonal communication that they later regretted. Chapters 2 and 3 discussed the biologic response that causes people to immediately respond or to defend their actions. (See **FIGURE 7.2**.) It is important for leaders to understand these responses, and it is advisable to read additional material (suggestions are included in the resources section at the end of the book). The key is to recognize an emotional surge as it is triggered and to allow it time to pass. Research has demonstrated that strong initial emotions last for approximately 90 seconds before they begin to dissipate. If a person stays emotionally charged up longer than 90 seconds, it is probably by choice.

What is valuable here is the realization that leaders have a choice about how they respond when they notice their automatic response has been triggered. If they are paying attention, and if they are especially attentive during situations that have caused anxiety and distress in the past, then they know when to expect the automatic response and they can allow themselves to watch as it passes, choosing instead to have curiosity and engage when they have developed a reasoned and diplomatic response.

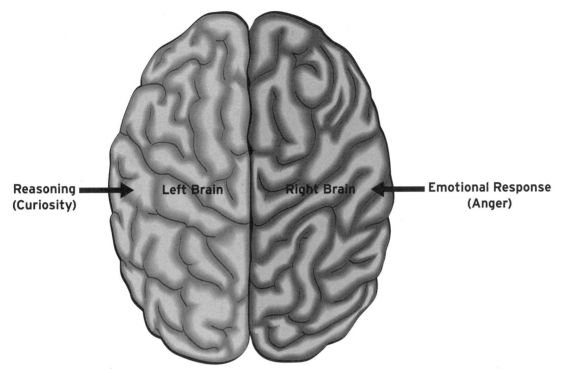

FIGURE 7.2 It is important for leaders to understand the biologic response that causes people to immediately respond or to defend their actions. The key is to recognize an emotional "surge" as it is triggered and to allow it time to pass.

Effective Followers

Leaders need followers. Being an effective follower is an art of its own, requiring many of the same basic behaviors as described earlier for leaders. The leadership/followership relationship is sustained when leaders meet followers' needs. Responsibility for the fulfillment of follower needs gives the leader the power of authority, whether the authority is positional or expert. Leaders are most effective if followers recognize the importance of maintaining key behaviors as part of a team:

- Mission safety is always a priority.
- Respect authority and act with integrity.
- Keep ego in check—attitudes are contagious.
- Respect others' opinions, views, and talents.
- Clearly articulate goals, skills, and tasks.
- Understand the limits of authority.
- Work to make the team successful.
- Do your part to maintain a safe environment for crew input.
- Acknowledge your own mistakes.
- Maintain your domain expertise—and keep learning.
- Keep the team briefed, and remain flexible.
- Communicate clearly, always stating your intent first.

Safe behaviors have to be consciously practiced. Loss of situational awareness has caused many injuries and deaths, and safety rules have been developed for a reason. A leader should not have to constantly remind followers about the importance of wearing seat belts, properly donning protective equipment, and practicing conscious awareness during routine tasks. Team and individual safety is always a priority, and also a responsibility. Consider the following case.

> **CASE STUDY 6**
>
> Fire Fighter William "Bull" Davis was a crusty veteran of 22 years and had always worked at Station 16 on Ladder 7, one of the busiest houses in the city. He was known for doing things his own way, and few new officers questioned his
>
> *(continues)*

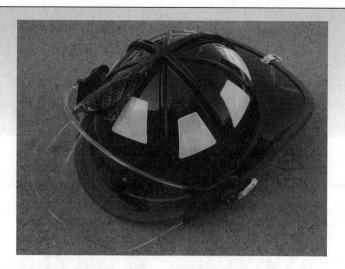

old-style methods and practices. When Lieutenant Frank Gett was promoted, he was assigned to Ladder 7 on "Bull" Davis's shift. Lieutenant Gett was a 12-year veteran who prided himself on staying abreast of the latest trends in firefighting safety and survival. After two months on the job at Ladder 7, Lieutenant Gett was tired of telling Fire Fighter "Bull" Davis to pull on his flame-resistant hood, fasten his seat belt, and move his helmet strap from the back of his helmet to under his chin where it belonged. Worse, Lieutenant Gett noticed that his other two fire fighters, one with 3 years of experience and the other with 5 years, were starting to emulate their old buddy Bull. After all, only newbies buckled their seat belts and used the strap on their helmets, according to Bull.

After getting no results with coaching and counseling, Lieutenant Gett started developing a paper trail on Bull, documenting his policy breaches and giving him corrective action, including once sending him home for the day. Shortly thereafter, Ladder 7 was sent to a greater alarm fire at the Alladin Hotel, a brick structure built in 1895 and remodeled several times since. During the fire, Ladder 7's crew was sent inside a rear staging area and ordered to cut the utilities to the building. Once inside and while engaged in securing the gas meter, the rear roof collapsed, trapping the crew from Ladder 7.

When all five members were finally pulled out, two had died from head trauma—fire fighter "Bull" Davis and the 3-year fire fighter. The subsequent investigation found that both fire fighters were found without their helmets, and both suffered from what was described as "survivable" traumatic injuries. In the case of Fire Fighter Davis, he had been knocked unconscious and subsequently died from smoke inhalation. His position was found to be "unencumbered," meaning had he been conscious, he could have crawled to safety.

The report was extremely critical of the crew's safety awareness, noting that three of the five members (including both fatalities) had their helmet chin straps buckled over the rear rim of their helmets. When Lieutenant Gett was questioned by the investigators, he mentioned how difficult it was to constantly stay aware of dynamic fireground situations while also attempting to consistently remind some crew members to follow simple safety rules, such as wearing fire-resistant hoods and securing their helmets by buckling their chin straps properly.

Distractions during a dynamic event, whether a resuscitation, fire, or hazardous materials incident, are to be expected. However, distractions that are caused by a failure to follow simple safety procedures are unacceptable and lead to an erosion of team safety. In addition, they also distract from the task at hand, which is constantly working to achieve a collective situational awareness related to the current incident.

Had Fire Fighter "Bull" Davis decided instead to use his experience and expertise in the role of a positive mentor, things would have been different. If that were the case, Lieutenant Gett would not have spent his workdays distracted by a follower who made his own rules and ignored safety, and he also would have had help in developing the new fire fighters. Additionally, it's likely that the two fire fighters would be alive today to tell their story.

Effective followers, through commitment to the leader and the mission, permit teams to achieve benchmarks and goals. Being a good follower is sometimes more difficult than being a good leader. Followers must accept the responsibility to stay mentally and physically fit, must maintain their area of expertise, must understand the strengths and weaknesses of their team members (including themselves), must maintain a positive attitude, and should regularly practice communication skills. They should recognize that as stress levels increase during a critical event, operational distraction is a risk that must be managed.

Because CRM is a tool that allows followers to challenge a leader's decision, the responsibility of followers to act appropriately is paramount. Proper conduct and acceptable group behavior are critical; without them, effective communication breaks down. Not even the most effective and calm leader can tolerate personal attacks or rude behavior, and followers can find themselves shut out of the discussion, regardless of how critical or pertinent their observations.

Challenging Decisions as an Effective Follower

Any challenge to a decision should be done in an assertive and respectful way. Earlier the methodology of **PACE** was described, or probing, alerting, challenging, and taking emergency interventions. It can be helpful for team members to practice different techniques for how to conduct themselves effectively in the CRM environment so that they become comfortable and learn to understand when to challenge and when to intervene. Assertive communication for followers involves the following steps, at a minimum:

1. Gain the person's attention. Say the person's name (or use rank if appropriate). Do not randomly query the entire team or make a general statement.
2. State your intent, your concern, and own your emotional response. For example: "Captain, my intent is to see whether you are aware of a potential safety problem. I feel uncomfortable with Plan A."
3. State the problem as you see it, whether real or perceived. For example: "I think the roof is unstable and could collapse."
4. Offer a proposed alternate action. For example: "We could initiate a defensive attack for a few minutes and see if we achieve knockdown."
5. Request feedback. For example: "What are your thoughts?"

It is important for team members to remember that the feedback may not be in agreement with their proposal. The benefit to open communication is *not* that everyone agrees with the challenger's specific course of action or idea, but that everyone within the team is aware of potential dangers and pitfalls. The goal is collective situational awareness and a shared understanding, not an approach that is completely cohesive.

In addition, one must be careful to use words that question the tactic or the objective, not the intelligence or motive of the person making the decision. Using language that is condescending or derogatory only serves to inflame the situation and may provoke a defensive response from leaders who do not fully understand how their ego or emotional response can affect their decision process. A leader who is defensive may be distracted and discount information, regardless of how important it is.

The root cause of communication failure between followers and leaders can often be traced to barriers caused by the perception of incompetence and loss of dignity. Any challenge that places the leader in a position where she loses dignity or her authority is eroded will have negative consequences for team performance and cohesiveness (not to mention the possibility of lingering resentment).

Whereas in nonemergency situations these challenges usually can be resolved by having a conversation in a private setting, that's not often possible during an emergency. If a team member believes he or she has used the respectful and assertive approach appropriately, but still receives a powerful defensive response from the team leader, it is important for him or her to follow up after the emergency and engage in discussions to clarify roles and responsibilities during emergency team operations. Reviewing the goals and objectives of CRM can be valuable. In particular, if the leader continues to place his or her team in danger regardless of how well the team is attempting to communicate, it is time for the team member to move up the hierarchy in expressing concerns. If this is necessary, it is critical that the team member first tell the team leader, and then use specific examples and express concerns in a way that indicates the team member is not conducting a personal attack but instead laying out behaviors that are endangering personnel. This is illustrated in the following case.

CASE STUDY 7

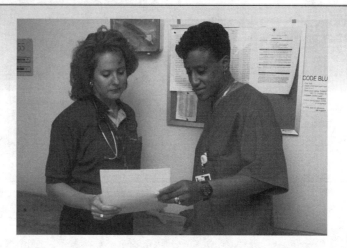

At Peace Harbor Trauma Center, Critical Care Registered Nurse (CCRN) Pam Gillete was proud of her role as the lead trauma nurse. A Level One Trauma Center, Peace Harbor regularly received patients by ground and by air from the surrounding community, which had a population of more than 2 million people. It was not uncommon to get between 8 and 10 trauma system patients per day, and there were two trauma teams on duty around the clock.

One team was regularly led by Dr. Pierce Nodaway, a skilled trauma surgeon who had developed his craft while working in forward-based hospitals in the military. He was known, however, for regularly ignoring the rules.

In 2007, the trauma center enacted policies that required a checklist approach to any patient admitted to the trauma service. It was particularly important to Pam that these checklists be followed because their development and use had come from a quality improvement process that followed four incidents where serious medical errors were made. Although she understood the reluctance of some veterans, like herself, she also knew that no clinician could remember everything, particularly under duress. Pam's insistence on the use of the checklists was especially robust with pediatric patients because their weight-based interventions could be particularly prone to error.

On four occasions in 2007 and another five in 2008, Pam noted that there were no checklists generated by Dr. Nodaway's trauma teams. When asked, the lead nurse on Dr. Nodaway's team said that he would refuse to use them and would often be critical of those team members who tried to do so. "Lists are for the incompetent," he once said.

Each time she noted the discrepancy, Pam approached Dr. Nodaway, and in her capacity as the lead trauma nurse in charge of trauma service quality told him that he needed to start using the tools provided. According to Pam's notations, Dr. Nodaway either ignored her or "humored" her by stating he would start using them right away.

Without making any character judgments, and without attacking his motives, Pam simply told him that she would be filing a request with the hospital clinical manager that Dr. Nodaway be removed from trauma service call. She used the specific examples of his behavior, noted that the rules were in place to minimize errors and injury, and also noted that everyone else, regardless of their level of experience, was using the checklists effectively.

Dr. Nodaway's complaints about being removed fell on deaf ears. Peace Harbor had a long history of innovation, safety, and teamwork, and the clinical manager recognized that her team and their commitment to effective leaders was the best defense she had against mistakes and errors.

Getting to Know the Team Leader

Leaders and followers should spend time getting to know each other, discovering each other's strengths, weaknesses, skills, and experiences. However, it is not always possible to do this on a personal level when teams are thrown together in an emergent situation. Even members of teams that have been together for a while can forget this important step. Leaders who understand the strengths of every follower are more successful in achieving team goals, and they also provide a safer environment with better decision making, and followers who know their team members well can capitalize on each other's strengths and compensate for any weaknesses.

For example, good "street" paramedics often are considered those who can quickly and decisively make decisions related to critical patient care. They operate on intuition and recognition-primed decision making rather than solely on protocol. In many ways, they trade accuracy for speed in a manner that might be necessary to intervene quickly and save a life. However, a response to a hazardous materials incident takes a different kind of expert. In these situations, a team's most methodical members are likely the most valuable. The step-by-step approach of cross-referencing materials from multiple sources and securing a scene before acting is more likely to lead to a successful outcome. In these situations, trading accuracy for speed would mean failing to follow each step, resulting in a wrong tactic and a potentially catastrophic outcome. Different teams need different skills and strengths and need to be treated differently. A one-size-fits-all approach will not bring leadership success.

Lifelong Learners

The most valuable followers in a team are the lifelong learners, those who are able to keep their ego in check and who strive to maintain and further develop their skill set. Followers who stay ahead of the learning curve in their specific domain have a deeper reservoir of options to draw from during an event. They better understand the pros and cons of a specific strategy. More important, they have stayed abreast of their craft by reading accounts of other incident successes and failures and by learning from those incidents, which might not yet have occurred in their agency.

Chapter 4 discussed the case of Gunther Foss, the unfortunate individual who tried to trim his tree next to high-voltage lines. During the discussion regarding rescue options, a local power company representative confirmed that an inline breaker had tripped, ensuring the power was off to the lines that were adjacent to the tree. This, of course, generated discussion around performing an immediate rescue of the individual. However, one of the command staff on scene stepped up and mentioned that he had recently taken a class on safe practices around power lines. Although the class was specific to fighting wildland fires, he stated that the power company can remotely reset the breakers and often sends a large surge of power through the lines immediately after reset in the hopes of "blowing off" any branches that might have come into contact with the line. Needless to say, this significantly changed the course of the discussion. It was a valuable contribution from someone who cared enough to continue perfecting his knowledge base and was open enough to share his knowledge with others.

Followers should also be prepared to keep the team and the team leader briefed on their assignment. In particular, it is important for the leader to know whether there are impediments to completing a certain task. It also builds team credibility and trust when followers freely and quickly admit any mistakes they might have made during the execution of their tasks. There is little room for a defensive or protective attitude within a successful dynamic team. If all members are focused on the objective, and if they all are working to make each other successful, communicating failures along with successes becomes a normal operational mode.

Good followers are flexible. Great planning does not always result in a great strategic victory. Often the best-laid plans are no match for Mother Nature or the rapid dynamic developments teams face with seriously injured patients or complex fire scenes. A flexible attitude is helpful, as is approaching incidents with the understanding that tactics and strategies will likely change. When this attitude is taken, rapid developments are less surprising.

Types of Follower Behavior

Like leaders, followers who are engaged in high-risk teams have been studied in many different circumstances. Researchers have noticed certain categorical types of behavior practiced by followers. Following are descriptions of these categorical behaviors:

- Sheep
- "Yes people"
- Alienated followers
- Effective followers

Dependent, Noncritically Thinking Followers

Followers who never question or contribute are known as sheep. Sheep are rarely active in the CRM process and don't provide the team with critical thinking abilities. They sit quietly on the side, showing up when told to (not before), conducting their vehicle and equipment checks, and going home when the duty shift is over. A sheep is not interested in contributing to the crew and offers nothing in an emergency. They tend to go along with any decision, good or bad. After the incident is over, they're standard response is, "I did what I was told to do."

Engaging sheep in a CRM process can be difficult. Often, in the person's history is an incident when the individual was criticized for speaking up. One of the strategies a leader can use to convert a sheep into an effective team member is to pull the person aside and express how important it is for the individual to participate. For example, if the person has a particular skill or domain experience, the leader can emphasize how the team will gain value from having the individual provide more effective input.

The sheep must know that the leader is creating a safe environment and that participation is welcome. If there is a past history of ill treatment, the leader should address that specifically and assure the person that he will do everything in his power to protect his team.

More dangerous on the crew are the "yes people" who make decisions based on whatever the leader says. These people may be far more engaged than the sheep in that they will often be in the forefront, right with the leader. They sometimes strive to be the "official deputy" of the leader and may gain a position on the team based more on their ability to befriend the right people than their technical skills or abilities. Their behavior and regular confirmation of the leader's direction can contribute to a homogenized way of thinking and may give the leader a false sense of security because a devil's advocate or worst-case-scenario position was never considered.

Although this behavior is often used to avoid conflict, it is certain to lead to groupthink-type situations, where collective situational awareness and regular updating do not occur. It is actually fairly easy for leaders to deal with this type of behavior. However, sometimes ineffective leaders purposefully surround themselves with these types of followers to minimize conflict and satisfy their ego.

Critically Thinking Followers

Critical thinking behaviors are reflected in the actions of both alienated and effective followers. **Alienated followers** are bright and critical thinkers, yet often withhold information because of anger or unresolved conflict with crew members or the leader. Alienated followers are often looking to destroy teamwork and should be removed unless the conflict can be resolved.

The danger of alienated followers is that they have a different commitment than the rest of the team. Instead of being committed to the mission and the team's success, they are often committed to proving themselves right. This behavior ensures that the story they are telling themselves (e.g., the organization is bad, these people are bad, I didn't get a chance and someone else did) will seem to be the accurate one.

Alienated followers are not hard to identify. They are often smart, well informed, and experienced. Their attitude, however, is usually readily apparent. They are not generally willing to step forward and take on responsibility, and they frequently avoid team communication opportunities. Removing them from the team can be difficult in that these people typically have a depth of experience and may be the only personnel on the team with specific expertise in a certain area. Leaders must evaluate whether they can manage the collateral damage caused by this person while valuing his or her input, whether they can turn the person around into a committed believer, or whether it is better to let the person go.

Effective followers are active without being "yes people" and are not afraid to speak up and challenge a decision. They exhibit several of the successful behaviors discussed previously and are constantly working to improve personal and team performance. Leaders can reward these individuals by giving them progressive responsibility. Team leaders should allow them to learn from their mistakes, expand their horizons, and at times, take them out of their comfort zone by offering them assignments that are not within their particular domain.

Poisonous Team Member Behaviors

Behaviors that can be specifically exhibited by those in leadership roles and those who are followers have been discussed, but it is also important to mention a few hazardous behaviors that any team member, leader or follower, can exhibit. Generally speaking, these hazardous behaviors cover most of the problematic issues that are identified when a bad incident occurs and the "human factor" investigation points to behavior problems (in earlier chapters, it was discussed that bad behavior is rarely a single contributing causal factor in accidents).

Annual fire and emergency medical services (EMS) accident reports list regular instances where individuals ignored good rules, acted impulsively and without the proper risk analysis, or elected to disregard safety procedures. **Table 7.1** describes antidotes for each of the following hazardous behaviors.

Antiauthority behavior can, in the right circumstances, be a constructive and refreshing experience. It is often how old ways of doing things are challenged and new procedures shaped. But team members must find the proper balance between respectfully challenging old rules that no longer make sense and disparaging good rules that are current, relevant, and in place for a reason. Most times, rules challenges should take place in a constructive manner and be associated with thought-provoking discussion—they should not occur during an emergent, dynamic incident. If a team member believes that the current rules don't apply, the individual often can engage in changing them. However, rules challengers should be prepared to conduct an analysis of the current best practices, should be able to discuss the situations when the rule must always be followed and the situations when rules may have to be modified, and need to agree on how the organization should follow up when it finds inaccurate or outdated rules and policies in place.

Although impulsive behavior is often attributed to inexperienced people, injury and death statistics demonstrate that anyone, regardless of experience, can be a victim of *impulsivity*. Unfortunately, those in the fire, EMS, and critical care industries have a tendency to act first on many occasions, mainly because of the time-compressed nature of their business. Certainly, in some situations sitting back to think things over will result in a life lost. However, the emergency nature of an individual's work doesn't mean that he must treat all situations as if they were emergencies. Often, waiting 10 seconds before responding can provide just enough of an edge in allowing the adrenalin rush to pass and the brain to engage.

When Paul LeSage first became a fire fighter, he had a veteran lieutenant named Earl. Earl was never impulsive. As a matter of fact, when Paul once asked him how he remained so calm on emergency scenes, he responded, "Well, that's not my stuff on fire." In thinking about Earl's response, it wasn't that he was callous, he had simply determined a method where he could remain calm and thoughtful, regardless of the chaos surrounding him. As a leader or a follower, impulsivity can be dangerous and counterproductive. A leader has demonstrated behavior that others will follow—the impulsive leader will have impulsive followers. For a follower, impulsive behavior can place them in danger by distracting the leader and other team members from their primary mission or objectives.

Another behavior that leaders and followers need to be aware of is *invulnerability*. For example, it's not hard for a new fire fighter to feel invulnerable after strapping on all the gear, helmet, fire-resistant clothing, and self-contained breathing apparatus (SCBA). With a good hose line, what can stop him? Invulnerable behavior manifests in small rule violations as well as large ones. It is seen in people who don't wear seat belts and who don't take the small but important safety precautions, such as wearing a reflective vest while working road incidents. Leaders can help thwart invulnerable behavior by

Table 7.1 Antidotes to Hazardous Behaviors

Hazardous Behavior	Antidote
Antiauthority "Don't tell me."	"Follow the rules. Work to change them if they are not right."
Impulsivity "Do something–quickly!"	"Not so fast. Think first."
Invulnerability "It won't happen to me."	"It can happen to me."
Machismo "I can do it."	"Taking chances is foolish."
Resignation "What's the use?"	"I'm not hopeless. I can make a difference in my world."
Pressing "Let's hurry up and get this thing done so that we can go home."	"If a job is worth doing, it is worth doing right the first time."
Air Show Syndrome "I am going to look so good. Look at me."	"Let's get the job done right by working as a team."

regularly using actual case scenarios to drive the point home: "There was nothing special about the last person who was injured or who died—he was another fire fighter, just like you. It can happen to you, too."

Machismo, or the "can-do" attitude, can be a great team-building behavior. Many teams pride themselves on their can-do attitude and are particularly competitive when it comes to specific skill sets, such as extrication. There is nothing wrong with instilling a sense of pride and ownership in a crew, and certainly nothing wrong with striving to be the best. However, there is a fine line between "can do" and "never done it, but will try anyway regardless of the risks." This behavior can go hand-in-glove with the feeling of invulnerability, and the behaviors are often seen together. When this behavior is being exhibited, it is important to clarify the objectives, ground the team in reality, and outline the risks associated with acting.

Resignation is a sign that a team member has given up. There can be many different reasons for this, but one of the most common is resistance to change. When individuals resist change, they develop an anxiety associated with their place, their skill sets, or their responsibilities. They may have received negative feedback or been introduced to something that appears overwhelming. Leaders can manage this behavior by pulling the individual aside and asking specific questions related to why the person is feeling resigned. Affirming the person's value to the team can be helpful, specifically if a leader can use examples of when the individual helped in the past or overcame other obstacles.

Pressing is a behavior that is extraordinarily common in emergency services. This is the trading accuracy and safety for speed behavior discussed earlier. Because the dominant mode while on scene or caring for a victim is one of action, team members tend to defer to the pressing mode for many other situations that actually might be better handled with a more measured approach. This is another behavior that, if exhibited by a team leader, will be mimicked by the followers. If the leader acts like things need to get done quickly, the followers will act the same way (maybe impulsively). On the other hand, when a team leader takes deliberate action to focus the team on doing the job well, evaluating the risks, and taking the proper safety precautions, it can help tone down the response of the followers.

The term **air show syndrome** or air show behavior has been used to define behavioral attributes that are associated with people who need to show off or demonstrate that they are better than others. Whether this behavior is associated with a need for attribution or to stoke their ego, it can be remarkably dangerous. Leaders need to specifically and directly address air show behavior when they see it, particularly if it involves violating safety norms, which it often does. In *Darker Shades of Blue: The Rogue Pilot*, an outstanding after-action analysis associated with the crash of a B-52 at Fairchild Air Force Base on June 24, 1994, Major Tony Kern describes this type of behavior. Kern outlines specific leadership failures that preceded the crash and that are instructive in any environment where operator safety is paramount.

Summary

Teams need leaders, and leaders need followers. Specific behaviors by leaders and followers contribute to successful teams and help foster open communication. In teams that are assigned critical, life-saving tasks, it is extremely important for team members to understand the qualities and skill sets of each member and to be able to help other members achieve maximum performance. Team members must be committed to the team and its mission, and leaders earn team member commitment through delegation, empathy, understanding, and mentoring.

Certain behaviors are risky, and both leaders and followers can fall into these behavior traps. It is everyone's responsibility to watch out for team members and to speak up if certain behavioral attributes place the team or individual members at risk.

Wrap Up

Ready for Review

- Good leaders desire a shared understanding among team members when it comes to mission goals and objectives. This common understanding can be promoted by the leader, by asking team members to restate specific goals or objectives.
- Leaders must be able to create situational awareness among team members, identify goals, and set specific and achievable objectives. Strong leaders will identify goals after first gaining a sense of what is happening at an incident scene and what needs to be done.
- Good leaders are expected to continually evaluate risk, which means they need to be ready to make adjustments at a moment's notice and listen carefully for indications that the current strategy may not be working.
- Absence of conflict is not what makes a good team. A good team understands how to resolve conflict and manage its potential effects, such as feelings of low self-esteem on the part of those involved in the conflict.
- The leadership/followership relationship is sustained by a leader meeting his or her follower's needs. The leader's power of authority comes from his or her responsibility for the fulfillment of those needs.
- The root cause of communication failure between followers and leaders can often be traced to barriers caused by the perception of incompetence and loss of dignity.

Vital Vocabulary

Air show syndrome Behavioral attributes that are associated with people who need to show off or demonstrate that they are better than others.

Alienated follower An alienated follower will withhold information due to anger or unresolved conflict with crew members or the leaders and are often looking to sabotage teamwork.

Mentor An individual with more experience in the domain, and often older, who helps guide another individual's professional and personal development.

PACE A method used to challenge team decisions in an assertive and respectful way; Probing, Alerting, Challenging, and taking Emergency Interventions.

Assessment in Action

1. Which behavior is not part of assertive communications with a leader?
   A. Gain the person's attention.
   B. State your intent, your concern, and own your emotional response.
   C. Threaten to document the encounter if the leader fails to listen.
   D. Offer a proposed alternate response to the problem as you see it.
2. Research has demonstrated strong, initial emotions last for approximately how long?
   A. 1 hour
   B. 90 seconds
   C. Years
   D. They can be controlled and avoided.
3. Conflict in a team environment is:
   A. destructive and should be avoided.
   B. usually attributed to one disgruntled team member.
   C. must be documented for disciplinary reasons.
   D. is a natural and predictable facet of team behavior.
4. Relationship management includes which of the following items?
   A. Diplomacy
   B. Protocols and SOPS
   C. Predatory behavior
   D. Contracts

In-Classroom Activity

1. Guide students through the five steps for mentoring, and have them prepare a document with which to approach a mentor:
   - Write down in descriptive terms specific areas where you need assistance.
   - Describe what you would like from a mentor.

- For each area in which you desire assistance, think about someone you respect in that particular domain and consider whether they will listen to you.
- Present your request to your future mentor with enough context for the person to understand your objective, your needs, and your concerns.
- Consider ahead of time what benefits you can offer to your mentor.

2. Have students role-play for a scenario in which Captain Albert confronts BC Gregory (from Case Study 4) about the deployment of more resources at the Orpheum Theater fire. Follow the CRM five-step model.
3. Conduct a group discussion to identify strategies for dealing with dependent, noncritically thinking followers, including sheep, "yes people," and alienated followers.

Reference

1. Anthony T. Kern, *Darker Shades of Blue: The Rogue Pilot*. (New York, NY: McGraw Hill, 1999).

8

Postincident Analysis

Objectives

- Describe the motivations for a postincident analysis.
- Describe the assumptions behind a postincident analysis.
- List the types of incidents that warrant a postincident analysis.
- Describe the techniques for conducting a formal postincident analysis.

CASE STUDY 1

As the Adams County helicopter Air-Rescue Six lifted off from the Pacific University helipad, Flight Paramedic/Deputy Sheriff Mike Harder felt the aircraft dip slightly to the left. At the same time, Pilot Jeff Reager moved the collective to the right as he felt a slight "tug" on the helicopter. Their flight recorder captured the conversation. "What the hell was that?" said Reager. "I'm not sure," replied Harder.

As Air-Rescue Six hovered for a moment above the pad, the dispatcher cleared them to head toward Highway 314, where a seriously injured patient was being extricated from a vehicle crash. Reager applied power and the aircraft gained altitude as it moved over the hospital parking lot. Suddenly, both Harder and Reager heard a loud "slapping" noise outside the helicopter. Something was banging on the left side of the aircraft. Harder twisted around

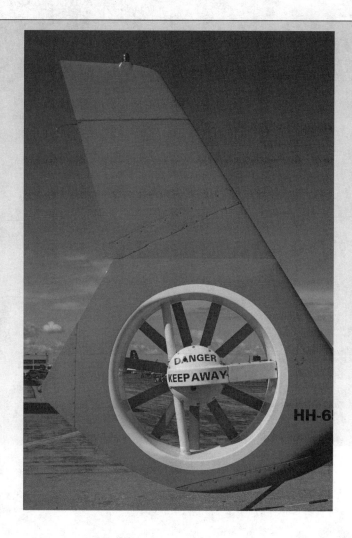

in his seat and prepared to crack open his door. "Door opening," he stated to Reager, and as he looked out, he reported, "Our power cord is still attached to the ship."

Jeff Reager slowed carefully and brought Air-Rescue Six to a safe landing on the expansive side lawn of the hospital. After canceling the mission through dispatch (mechanical problems), he shut down the Eurocopter EC-135 and both men climbed from the cockpit. Reager later reported "feeling sick" as he saw the 50-ft (15.2-m) extension cord wrapped several times around the aircraft's tail boom. Only the fact that the EC-135 had an enclosed tail rotor had kept the cord from becoming entangled in the rear rotor, which would have almost certainly led to a hard landing or a crash. The 50-ft (15.2-m) power cord was a "land-line" between the aircraft and a 110-volt power outlet on the helipad. The constant power allowed the crews to keep medical equipment charged while the helicopter sat idle. It generally was considered the paramedic's responsibility to remove the cord prior to flight, but the pilot also had a preflight checklist he was supposed to use that ensures the cord has been disconnected.

During the postincident analysis, Reager and Harder discovered that this was actually the third time such an event had happened in the past 36 months. Although the other events had generated internal investigations, the situations had never been debriefed and the lessons were never shared among all crew members.

Harder and Reager wrote an article about their experience, and they also initiated a process where all near-miss and unusual events were debriefed. The **debriefing** was first done with the involved crew and flight line staff, and then with the entire group so that everyone could learn.

A debriefing allows members who were involved to speak up in a nonthreatening environment and brings out issues that can be collectively discussed so that common resolutions can be found. Although such a debriefing doesn't guarantee that another similar incident will not occur, the debriefing process has been proven to embed lessons learned in an organization.

Quite often, an observer can determine what type of learning occurred in an organization by how the organization handles communications and quality improvement after a major response or a critical call. The attention that senior leaders give **postincident analysis (PIA)** and debriefing determines how seriously the organization embraces learning and quality improvement, as does the attitude with which PIA is completed. (See **FIGURE 8.1**.) A postincident analysis is an activity involving command and response personnel, taking place after an incident response. It reviews performance of individuals and teams, while focusing on learning lessons that can be applied to future incidents.

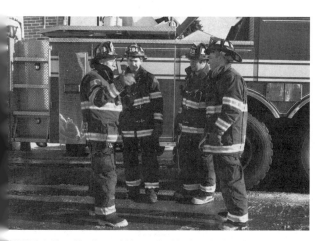

FIGURE 8.1 The attention paid to postincident analysis determines how seriously the organization embraces learning and quality improvement.

Motivations for Postincident Analysis

In nonlearning organizations, when things go right on an incident response, the responders usually don't see a reason to discuss the incident from a critical perspective. When things go wrong, however, responders are eager to participate in a critical review for several reasons, including placing blame, exposing incompetence, or watching someone "get what they deserve." This behavior is learned and is fairly common in emergency service organizations. After all, why would a team get together unless it was "to get chewed out by the battalion chief" for instance?

In a learning organization, leaders realize that opportunities to critique and improve performance in a positive environment are a gift. Teaching leaders and followers to appreciate this gift and not abuse it can be difficult. Because of busy schedules and crews that are spread out in a large system, most organizations don't support group communication after responses until an event of significance occurs. Many policies related to conducting PIAs specifically direct that they occur only after large-scale incidents, such as multiple-alarm fires, mass casualty incidents, or situations that resulted in damage or injury. These big incidents, by their very nature, are replete with operational mistakes and errors of every size. However, teams don't learn well if all they study are the large-scale events.

Learning organizations take advantage of the day-to-day incident volume and the small operational opportunities that they encounter. The leaders know that it is easier to pay attention to the details during smaller events, where there are fewer distractions. If the lessons learned can be shared openly afterward in a PIA environment, field operations personnel are more likely to perform better and make fewer mistakes when the "big one" occurs.

Additionally, it is important that midlevel managers who conduct debriefings be trained in the craft. Expecting a battalion chief who has the demeanor of a pit bull to successfully extract confessions related to errors made from a group of fire fighters is a stretch.

Ultimately, the motivations for performing postincident analysis should focus on improving communications, performance, and behavior and correcting inefficiencies for the benefit of future responses. An open and inviting atmosphere with a nonpunitive theme is most important. If there is a whiff of fear or retribution in the room, a leader can declare game over because participants will not participate openly and positive learning will not occur. It is also helpful to remind the group about their responsibility to speak up in their team. Using the crew resource management (CRM) loop, leaders should ask participants to point out areas where better communication may have helped or where changing strategies could have affected the outcome.

Assumptions Behind Postincident Analysis

Performing a well-planned PIA for a specific incident can be time consuming and laborious and requires excellent **PIA facilitator** skills. A facilitator oversees the process of leading participants through a reconstruction of events, actions, and procedures that occurred during a response to an incident, with the outcome of improving future performance. A well-conducted PIA can also be a spontaneous, relaxed, professional airing of issues after what is considered a normal incident. Leader or facilitator skills are taught and learned; for most emergency responders they don't come naturally. Patience, group communication skills, and conflict resolution skills are critical to the process, and practice helps. Consider the following case study.

> **CASE STUDY 2**
>
> It was hot and uncomfortable in the summer afternoon following the annual disaster drill at the local airport. The emergency manager was conducting a PIA with about 120 people and eight agencies. The drill had produced the usual failures in individual and group communications: lack of interagency cooperation, untrained fair weather responders, and unclear response expectations, to name a few.
>
> As the two evaluators talked to each other in the background, predictable comments came from the fire fighters: "Well, he's going to go off on everybody about how badly they performed." "Watch the rookies cringe; they won't be back next year." "It will take years for the hard feelings to go away between the response groups." "Heaven forbid they have to respond to a real event." "I can't wait till next year."

In reality, the enmity of this situation started long before the disaster drill because most of the group behavior was a repeat from previous drills. Note that the first opportunity these agencies took to conduct a debriefing was after a complex, highly charged, multiagency drill where communications can be difficult even in the best of circumstances. This is why conducting mini PIAs after normal events is so helpful. The individuals involved are not under undue stress, the relationships are usually more secure, and the concept of discussing performance from a learning perspective can be introduced by a team leader in the spirit of building everyone's skill level.

Unfortunately, emergency responders are quite hard on themselves and their peers. It is the nature of the business for responders to be competitive, self-confident, and very direct in their actions. They often believe any scene that doesn't go right must be a failure and that someone is to blame.

Operator expectations of perfect incident response and performance are not realistic. When asked, most veteran responders will admit that they have never been to a perfect scene. In reality, there are too many variables and unknowns for responders to ever do tasks perfectly. It can be helpful to consider that someone else lost control of his or her world before calling for help and emergency responders use that as a starting point.

Tailboard Debriefings

Unfortunately, doing a full-blown PIA for every single response is not feasible. Usually, there isn't the time and opportunity to gather responders and incident detail together for every event. However, organizations can ensure that many calls are debriefed using the concept of the *tailboard debriefing* where the team leader, the company officer or senior emergency medical service (EMS) provider, assembles the crew around the tailboard of an engine, the back of the ambulance, on the helipad, or in the emergency department and reviews the call. Every scene should get a **hot wash**, in which responders can defuse the emotional charge of the scene, identify deficiencies and ineffective behaviors, and off-load any stress before the next event. A hot wash is a meeting of all responding personnel on a scene to participate in an informal debriefing of the events of the incident, actions taken, and problems encountered.

Importantly, someone should take the responsibility to write down the key points or lessons learned an rward them to the people who are responsible for quality improvement and training. A learning organization will trend these inputs and track them by category so that training can be designed to address specific areas where operators are having difficulty.

Consider the following example: Tualatin Valley Fire & Rescue (TVF&R) has developed a system for tracking the lessons learned that are collected from PIAs and from informal tailboard debriefings. First, typically the senior EMS or incident command (IC) officer on scene leads the debriefings. These leaders start by outlining their own performance, what they could have done better, what they missed, and what they think went well. They then ask for direct, specific feedback. What do the other team leaders think? What did they see and hear? How could the IC have done things differently?

After this, each team leader checks in with his team members and they roll through the same basic issues. By the time the group has finished, everyone has a collective understanding of their performance—the good, the bad, and the ugly.

Once the personnel return to quarters, the senior paramedic or battalion chief (depending on the incident type) e-mails the team leaders who were present at the on-scene debriefing and asks them to briefly make a note of their observations. These are copied to the organization's quality improvement team, which collects them into trend files that are used for further analysis and scenario-based training. (See **FIGURE 8.2**.)

Structure Fire Trend File: 2008 (Partial)

Situation - Event	Incident	Reference Number
FF injured wearing wrong gloves	080014567	122
5" hose trapped during lay-in by hand bar	080014567	123
800 radio failure in stairwell	080014583	144
Failure to conduct PAR after withdraw	080014583	145
FF injured wearing wrong gloves	080014627	149
Failure to get CARA report: extended Ops	080014627	150
Thermal imager failure during fire attack	080015604	166
FF burned on hand during fire attack	080015604	167
FF hand injury: laceration	080015776	173
Confusion regarding "A" side of structure	080015779	174
Company worked until low air alarm	080015894	188
Company failure to give CARA report	080016642	203
Near Miss: 4 FF under porch roof collapse	080016642	204
Near Miss: SCBA regulator failure	080017237	211
Thermal imager failure during roof Ops	080017432	214
FF hand injury during rescue Ops	080017544	218
Near Miss: backing incident/Engine	080017544	219
PAR conducted after withdraw, no tones	080018542	226
Company worked until low air alarm	080018542	227
800 radio failure during fire attack	080018659	233
Failure to acknowledge 10-minute timer	080018659	234

To see whether event was immediately referred to Safety, Health, and Survival Program, Training Division, or Logistics please see Reference File.

For full report on times and units on scene, refer to CAD Incident Report.

For more event details, refer to Reference File.

FIGURE 8.2 Sample trend file.

Learning organizations continually mine their experiences for information that can be used to improve performance. Organizations that do not continually mine for improvement data experience uncorrected attitudes, unresolved conflicts, and no opportunity for retraining before the next event. In emergency response systems, the cumulative stress that builds within personnel who do not have the opportunity to learn from their own performance and that of their peers can result in them continuing to make the same mistakes and errors, which will negatively affect attitudes and morale. It is better for personnel to off-load the stress and correct smaller deficiencies, rather than have it all come out at the "big one." Hot washes also provide a defined time and place to coach people for quality improvement and to reinforce the expectation that they will be held accountable, in a timely way, for performance on the preceding event.

Many organizations regularly miss these opportunities to discuss immediate past performance and instead rely on mechanisms such as annual performance appraisals to accomplish individual improvement. It is not constructive for a team member to receive a comment like "I didn't like your attitude on the scene of the car crash six months ago" at an annual meeting with his or her supervisor. Such comments are nearly impossible for personnel to respond to or learn from. To avoid such useless comments leaders at learning organizations take every opportunity to conduct PIAs, analyze daily performance, and make small course corrections on a regular basis. These are easier for team members to accept, and both leaders and followers can enhance their working relationships and their critical scene performance by addressing issues as they arise.

An effective team leader should be supportive during incidents, be empathetic to followers regarding any operational errors, and help the team review the incident (including any relevant protocols and practices) immediately afterward when things are fresh in the team's mind.

Types of Incidents That Warrant a PIA

Because it is not feasible to conduct a PIA for every single activity, it is helpful to prioritize incidents that need a PIA. It can be more valuable to review the smaller incidents than the larger ones because mistakes are "expected" to occur during multijurisdictional, major events. (See **FIGURE 8.3**.) Mistakes are not typically expected and are less tolerated in the day-to-day incidents, such as extrications and cardiac arrests. Here is a list of reasonable candidates for PIA:

- A structure fire with a multiple-unit response
- Any incident that an unusual event occurs: explosion, collapse, community violence

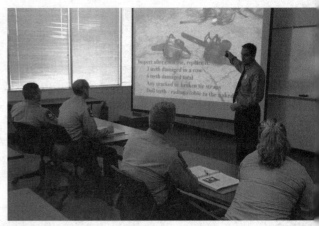

FIGURE 8.3 It can be more valuable to review the smaller incidents than the larger ones because mistakes are "expected" to occur during multijurisdictional, major events.

- Any incident resulting in a fatality or unusual human suffering (particularly if the victim is a child, a fellow emergency responder, or a family member)
- Any incident resulting in injury to an emergency responder
- Any close call where a responder could have been injured
- Hazardous materials incidents
- Mass casualty incidents
- Any incident involving multiple agencies
- Special operations incidents
- Mass gathering events: presidential visit, parades, large outdoor events
- Disaster drills and multiagency responses
- Emergency preparedness incidents such as natural or man-made disasters
- Incidents requiring conflict management/resolution between response groups

Techniques for Conducting a Formal PIA

Use of formal PIAs as an organizational learning tool shou[ld] be embedded in the fabric of the organization. All membe[rs] should recognize that an important goal is for the organiza[] tion to continually evolve and for personnel to contin[ue] to improve performance in their public service missio[n.] If individual and group performance is not reviewed fro[m] a learning perspective, improvement will be stagnant an[d] poor practices will become common practice. The follow[] ing is a guide for preparing for a formal PIA:

1. **Gather data and facts during the hot was[h] while they are still fresh.** Information su[ch] as run reports, scene diagrams, dispatch info[r] mation or tapes, and statements from respon[d] ers help reconstruct the event at the PIA. A[ny] details that help paint the picture of the eve[nt]

are valuable. Hearsay and conjecture are not admissible in this process and will derail and damage the PIA.
2. **Select the correct moderator/facilitator for the PIA.** As stated earlier, not all people have the ability to conduct a relaxed, participative, and nonpunitive PIA. It may be best to involve a facilitator who was either not directly involved in the situation or is considered neutral to conduct the event. If there is conflict between the facilitator and the personnel involved in the response incident, open communication and organizational learning will be hampered.
3. **Choose the time and place of the PIA.** Being timely with the PIA is important because personnel memories and interest in the event fade quickly. The PIA should be held within a few days of the response so that any ideas for improvement, conflict resolution, and getting on with the business of the department are delivered in a timely manner when the incident is fresh in responders' minds. Leaders should strive to gather most personnel involved in the event in a comfortable, neutral place and should place no time constraints on the meeting.
4. **Involve the relevant participants.** The personnel who participated in the original event, supervisory people, and support people should attend the event. The facilitator should be aware of nonparticipants and their influence on the activity. If disingenuous and extraneous personnel attend the PIA, the process will suffer. The PIA is not a media or circus event; it is a time for people to communicate, share, and improve. Many a PIA has turned into a witch hunt by having the wrong people present.
5. **Reconstruct the event.** It is the facilitator's responsibility to keep up the tempo of the meeting and guide the process of reconstructing the event. Using the diagrams, pictures, dispatch info, and run reports as references, the facilitator and key personnel can begin to tell the story. It is key to involve the actual on-scene personnel in recalling the sequence of events. (See **FIGURE 8.4**.) If the atmosphere of the event is supportive and positive, most responders will freely admit their mistakes and discussion on improvement can occur. If no one is opening up, the facilitator can coach them to do so and evaluate whether they have been damaged by previous PIA attempts.
6. **Deal with deficiencies.** If a few mistakes were made at the event and the group was able to flesh them out in a nonpunitive way during the PIA, the next step is to decide how to resolve the mistakes.

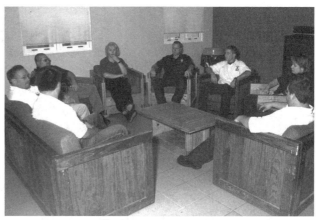

FIGURE 8.4 The facilitator is responsible for maintaining a supportive and positive atmosphere, while leading on-scene responders through postincident analysis. He or she should ask on-scene personnel key questions in order to reconstruct the incident: "When did you arrive?" "What was your task?" "What would you do differently?"

Facilitators should try to define the *nature* of the mistakes: Were they *system errors* (outdated, incomplete, or nonexistent policies, procedures, or practices), *education and training deficiencies*, *circumstances beyond the operators' control* (such as weather, crowds, and equipment breakage), or *human factors* (distractions, cognitive errors, or fatigue)? Infrequently, *behavioral issues* may have occurred. Behavioral problems are not errors or mistakes; they result from an operator's conscious choice to act, or behave, in a manner that is destructive, mean, or abusive. In the rare instances when a person's behavior was unacceptable and contributed to the poor outcome, team leaders may need to take corrective action with that person, which should never be done in a group setting. Otherwise, once leaders have defined the nature of the deficiencies, the group can pursue a method to fix the problems.

It is important to remember that the focus of the PIA is on learning, improving, and implementing solutions—not fixing blame.

Tools for PIAs

In a PIA, the following tools can be used to help with fact finding and to make analyses more consistent and complete:
- **PIA standard operating guidelines (SOGs):** Standard operating guidelines define using PIA as a part of departmental procedures and specify the who, what, when, where, and why of the process. They also institutionalize PIA as a highly desirable activity for the organization. **FIGURE 8.5** provides sample SOGs.

Lubbock Fire Department
General Procedures
Records and Reports
Postincident Analysis Program

I. PROCEDURES

    A. Formal Postincident Analysis

        1. 2nd alarm and specialty team response emergencies.
            a) All LFD personnel that participated in the emergency shall be required to attend the PIA if they are scheduled for duty that shift.
            b) Administrative, training, dispatch and FMO staff personnel that participated in the emergency shall be required to attend the PIA if they are scheduled for duty that day.

                (1) At least 24 hours notice should be given to staff personnel about the scheduled PIA.

        2. 3rd alarm or higher emergencies.
            a) Branch, division and group commanders that participated in the emergency shall be required to attend the PIA if they are scheduled for duty that shift.

                (1) They IC may require attendance of individual company officers based upon their response to the PIA questionnaire form.

            b) Staff personnel that participated in the emergency shall be required to attend the PIA if they are scheduled for duty that day.

                (1) At least 24 hours notice should be given to staff personnel about the scheduled PIA.

        3. Company officers shall complete the PIA questionnaire and email to the incident commander (IC) before the end of the shift that the incident occurred.
            a) The facilitator should review these questionnaires prior to the conducting of the PIA.

        4. The IC shall serve as the facilitator for the PIA.
            a) The IC is responsible for initiation of the formal PIA.

                (1) The formal PIA shall take place at the LFD training academy.

                (2) This PIA should not exceed 1 to 1 1/2 hours in length.

            b) The IC may make arrangements with the training academy for a facilitator to manage the PIA that was not involved in the incident.

                (1) These arrangements should be made at least 24 hours before the scheduled PIA.

            c) The IC shall notify and invite outside agencies and departments that may have responded to the incident to the PIA.
            d) This PIA should take place within 72 hours of the incident.

        5. The IC shall appoint a scribe to record points of discussion of major importance, recommendations, or suggestions as to possible solutions for problems encountered.
            a) The scribe should not be chosen from among the officers involved in the incident.

        6. The LFD PIA worksheet shall be utilized to guide and document the discussion.

FIGURE 8.5 Sample standard operating guidelines for a formal postincident analysis.

Source: Adapted from Lubbock Fire Dept. (Lubbock, TX) *Postincident Analysis Program*, 2002.

- Incident fact sheet: The incident fact sheet (see **FIGURE 8.6**) is a document in the PIA SOGs that assists responders with capturing key elements of the incident including the following:
1. Introduction
2. Building structure/site layout (use separate paper if more space is needed)
3. Fire code history
4. Communications
5. Pre-emergency planning
6. On-scene operations
7. Staging
8. Support functions
9. Safety group
10. Accountability
11. Investigations
12. Lessons learned
13. Overall analysis of incident

CASE STUDY 3

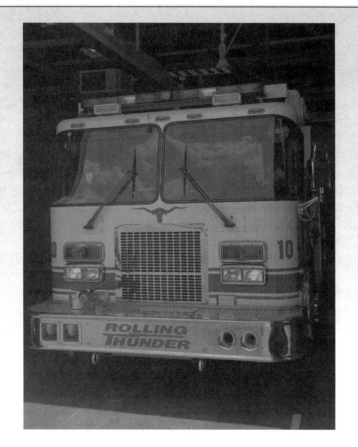

A midday response to an attached garage fire elicited a typical first alarm dispatch of two engines, one truck, one utility squad, and a battalion chief. The first arriving engine established command and spotted in front of the fully involved garage containing two vehicles. The second engine, arriving in two minutes, was directed to catch a hydrant and bring a water supply. The first engine crew pulled a preconnect attack line and advanced toward the fire, but the engineer was unable to charge the hose line because the pump would not engage.

This type of fire was not common for this department, so the stress level for all responders was quite high and only elevated by a large public gallery. An assistant chief happened to be riding with the first-in engine and observed the engineer trying to solve the problem with the pump engagement. As a

(continues)

result of this challenge, the IC ordered the second arriving engine to attack the fire upon arrival.

The fire was extinguished without incident, and salvage, overhaul, and restoration were also performed. In the hours following the event, the engineer on the first engine received lots of negative attention, some directly from superiors not present on the fire ground and some from other stations and personnel across the department. The criticism ranged from suggestions of incompetence, to retraining, to dismissal because the engineer was not able to get water from the first arriving engine. Unfortunately, these can be typical responses to a negative event unless personnel in the organization have been taught to manage the way stories are created, especially stories that are largely inaccurate, incomplete, harmful, and hurtful. (See Chapter 2 for more on organizational story and culture.)

The battalion chief scheduled a PIA for the next duty shift, two days later. No hot wash was conducted at the scene, but the battalion chief was able to conduct fact finding to a reasonable degree. The department mechanic checked out the apparatus and found nothing abnormal with the pump shift mechanism on the engine.

During the PIA, the captain on the first arriving engine detailed the difficulty they had in getting through traffic and that several grid-lock situations occurred and the air horn was use to clear the way. The captain had been newly promoted and admitted to being overexcited because this was his first fire as officer-in-charge. During the review of the engineer's performance, the assistant chief observed that correct procedures were followed by the engineer in trying to engage the pump.

The department head mechanic was present at the PIA and picked up the fact that the excessive use of the air horn may have dropped the stored air pressure tank to a point where the air-operated pump shift would not work.

The rest of the PIA was unremarkable, with a few comments on better spotting of apparatus. Subsequent testing to reenact the air horn use on this incident revealed that indeed the air tank pressure dropped below a level that would operate the pump shift mechanism, a new discovery for the department.

Suggestions from the PIA were based on evaluating the pump shift problem and educating other members on how to avoid this in the future. This event was caused by a combination of education and training deficiencies (no understanding of what would occur with overuse of the air horn) and a circumstance beyond the operator's control (pump won't engage in low air pressure tank situation). Recommendations included these:

- Department-wide training on air horn use that focuses on cause and effect (education and training approach)
- Installation of an air monitoring gauge for the engineer on the apparatus to monitor the air pressure of the air tank (system approach)
- Coaching of all department members to not speculate on individual performance, especially in the absence of facts (human factor approach)

The engineer, who was judged as a grade A performer for the organization, eventually chose to move to a different organization as a result of the unwarranted criticism for his performance.

Telegraph Fire Incident Fact Sheet
Managed by CAL FIRE and Incident Command Team 8,
Mariposa County Sheriffs Department,
and the Mariposa County Fire Department.

Date Updated: 7/29/08 Time: 7:00 AM

Fire Name: Telegraph **Start Date:** 7/25/2008 @ 3:10 PM **Cause:** Target shooting
Geographic Location: Mariposa, Greeley Hill, Midpines, Briceburg
Acres: 29,600 (46 sq mi.) **% Containment:** 10 **Estimated Containment Date:** Unknown
Cost to Date: $9,096,147.00 **Injuries:** 5 **Injuries to Date:** 9

Current Threats: Communities of Mariposa, Midpines, Greeley Hill, Coulterville, El Portal, Morman Bar, and Boot Jack. Mt. Bullion Conservation Camp, the Mariposa Utility District water supply, 70 kv transmission line supporting Yosemite Valley, as well as Yosemite National Park and numerous communication/repeater towers.

Current Road Closures: Highway 140 will be closed between the hours of 8:00 AM and 9:00 PM subject to change at any time 3 miles west of Briceburg and 4 miles west of El Portal at Cedar Lodge.

Evacuations: A mandatory evacuation for the Midpines Community is in effect. An evacuation advisory is in effect for all residences in the immediate fire area; which includes communities east of North Highway 49 at Mykleoaks Road south to the Highway 140 junction. This also includes communities west of Highway 140 from Mariposa north to Briceburg.

Evacuation Center: Mariposa Elementary School – 5044 Jones Street, Mariposa.

Animal Evacuations: Contact the animal evacuation hotline at 209-966-3615.

Structures Destroyed: Residence: 25 Outbuildings: 27 Residence Threatened: 4000

Difficulties in Control: Steep terrain, access, heavy and dry vegetation, high temperatures, low humidity.

Cooperating Agencies: CHP, Merced County Sheriff, Mariposa SPCA

Current Situation: The fire is making major runs in all directions through thick stands of manzanita, chamise, and oak. Extreme fire behavior was observed with flame lengths of up to 100 feet reported. Similar burning conditions are expected in the next 24 hours. The fire is moving into the Sierra and Stanislaus Forest, affecting 70 kv transmission line providing power to Yosemite Valley. A firing operation in the Dogtown area may generate visible smoke over the next 24 hours.

Resources Assigned: Engines: 408 Fire Crews: 71 Water Tender: 30 Dozers: 59
Helicopters: 13 Air Tankers: 6 Total Personnel: 3458

FIGURE 8.6 Sample incident fact sheet.

Courtesy of the California Department of Forestry & Fire Protection.

Idiosyncrasies of PIA

PIA must mirror the incident type (that is, fire, EMS, or law enforcement); one size does not fit all situations. Other aspects such as critical stress management must be taken into consideration when conducting a PIA following a critical incident. By definition, a critical incident is one that overwhelms the ability of a responder to cope with the experience, either at the scene or later. It has become standard practice for emergency response systems in the United States and abroad to deploy specially trained teams to conduct **critical incident stress debriefings (CISDs)**, confidential peer group discussions with personnel who have been involved in particularly traumatic calls or other painful incidents. A CISD is usually held within 24 to 72 hours of the incident. When extreme emotion is present, certain individuals may need to be referred to the employee assistance program or professional counseling.

At the beginning of each PIA session, the group must agree on behavior to be used in the analysis. Facilitators may challenge the group to accept a social agreement that includes listening with respect to others, allowing what goes on in the room to stay in the room, and reinforcing that with honesty comes amnesty within the group.

Summary

Postincident analyses and debriefings are crucial to organizations that want to learn from their everyday performance. Additionally, these exercises allow individuals to learn from their own mistakes and from the mistakes of others, and to use lessons learned to promote future proficient practices.

In PIAs, leaders step up and take responsibility for their own performance and for the performance of their followers. Leaders can gain commitment in their team by standing up and pointing out better ways of doing business, particularly if they allow their own decisions and actions to be reviewed. (See **FIGURE 8.7**.)

Learning organizations memorialize the lessons learned from an event so that operators do not repeat the same mistakes. They trend the types of errors and mistakes that are being made, and also the areas of excellence, so that training and quality improvement personnel can build programs that can have a powerful impact on safety and operational performance.

The most effective PIAs are structured so that each team member involved in the incident has time to speak and present observations. PIAs are conducted in an environment of safety. The facilitator must make it clear that no organizational stories are to be constructed from individual remarks and behaviors.

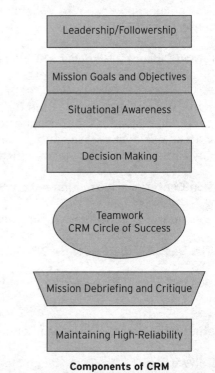

Components of CRM

FIGURE 8.7 Effective leadership is guided by a commitment to team mission goals and objectives. A good leader will place importance on each member's experience and observations by encouraging participation at PIAs. When situational awareness is maintained among the group, a team may efficiently evaluate and update standard procedure in order to maintain high reliability.

Wrap Up

Ready for Review

- Use of a formal PIA as an organizational learning tool should be embedded in the fabric of a CRM organization. All team members should recognize that an important goal of the organization is to continually evolve and improve performance in their public service mission.
- Performing a well-planned PIA for a specific incident can be time-consuming and laborious. It requires excellent facilitator skills. A well-conducted PIA can also be a spontaneous, relaxed, professional airing of issues after an incident.
- Every scene should get a hot wash, which is equivalent to a defusing on the scene that identifies and makes plans to improve deficiencies and behaviors. It also serves to off-load any stress on the part of the responders before they are called to the next incident.
- Operators often have unrealistic expectations for perfect incident response and performance. When asked, most veteran responders will say they have never been to a "perfect" scene.
- PIAs and debriefings are crucial, in that they allow organizations to learn from everyday performance. PIA activities also allow individuals to learn from their own mistakes and from the mistakes of others. Team leaders should use lessons learned during PIA to promote future proficient practices.

Vital Vocabulary

Critical incident stress debriefing (CISD) A confidential peer group discussion in which specially trained teams work with personnel who have been involved in traumatic calls or other painful incidents; CISDs usually occur within 24 to 72 hours of the incident.

Debriefing Allows members who were involved in an incident to speak up in a non-threatening environment, to bring out issues that can be collectively discussed and resolved.

Hot wash A meeting of all responding personnel on scene to participate in an informal debriefing of the events of the incident, actions taken, and problems encountered.

PIA facilitator An individual who oversees the process of leading participants through a reconstruction of events, actions, and procedures that occurred during a response to an incident, with the outcome of improving future performance.

Postincident analysis (PIA) An activity involving command and response personnel, taking place after an incident response. It reviews performance of individuals and teams, while focusing on learning lessons which can be applied to future incidents.

Assessment in Action

1. Debriefings should:
   A. include responders not present at the incident.
   B. serve as an opportunity to discipline individuals.
   C. be conducted by an experienced facilitator.
   D. be rigidly organized.
2. PIA:
   A. should include documentation of the incident and PIA activities.
   B. is required by OSHA.
   C. should involve senior officers not involved in the event.
   D. should involve mental health workers.
3. A punitive environment in a PIA:
   A. is proper for the activity.
   B. will shut down open communication among participants.
   C. must be documented, to discipline participants.
   D. will help to control the activity.
4. A learning organization uses critiques, such as PIA, to:
   A. document OSHA violations.
   B. enforce the chain of command.
   C. evaluate cost-effective strategies.
   D. develop open communication and learn from events.

In-Classroom Activity

Develop a short response scenario. The National Fire Fighter Near-Miss Reporting system is an excellent source of inspiration. You can access this resource at *www.firefighternearmiss.com*. Allow students to role-play the positions of facilitator, responder, and documenter in a postincident analysis. Ask students to prepare a list of actions to improve future performance and safety at a similar event.

9

Maintaining High Reliability

Objectives

- Define the term high-reliability organization.
- Describe the importance of mindfulness in maintaining safety.
- Describe how mindlessness leads to accidents.
- Describe how to assess the ability to inquire, doubt, and update.
- Describe the dangers to the team when there is a preoccupation with failure.
- Describe the importance of a reluctance to simplify.
- Describe how to build a commitment to resilience.
- Describe why deference to expertise is necessary.

CASE STUDY 1

On September 8, 2008, at 9:20 PM, Battalion Chief Roberto Olivio watched with satisfaction as the heavy black smoke pouring from the back of the building started to turn gray, then white. The Colony Apartments were older, built in 1974, and were not equipped with sprinklers, allowing a simple back deck fire to extend into the attic and burn across three units. Olivio had called a second alarm, bringing the total number of units on scene to eight engines, two trucks, one heavy rescue, and one safety officer in addition to himself and some folks from the Fire Investigations Bureau.

North Valley Fire Engine 118 and Ladder 83 had been first on scene, and Olivio observed that they would likely be one of the last to leave, based on their position at the front of the structure. Once the fire had been contained and overhaul started, BC Olivio started releasing crews to return home. In the postincident investigation, Olivio mentioned that he regretted not keeping a few more units on scene to help in the final overhaul, since he knew the crews from Engine 118 and Ladder 83 were tired.

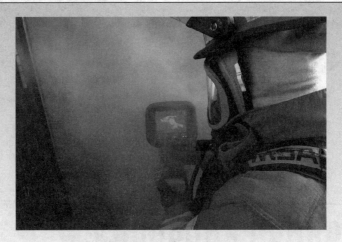

Once the scene was secured, Olivio turned it over to the investigators and the last of the fire fighters returned to their stations. A total of six units had been damaged or destroyed, and the entire fire building was vacated as a result.

At 1:33 AM on September 9, 2008, Olivio awoke to the sound of his fire pager. He recognized the address on the screen: it was the Colony Apartments. As he responded, dispatchers reported that the original fire building was heavily involved, and that fire had spread to the adjacent apartments where four people were reportedly trapped on a second-floor balcony.

Battalion Chief Olivio ordered a second alarm, and again Engine 118 and Ladder 83 were first on scene. Crews from both units rescued all four trapped residents, but the company officer on Ladder 83 was seriously injured when he fell from a 36-ft (11-m) ground ladder while getting ready to perform a primary search. After the second fire, an investigation showed that the original fire had not been completely extinguished and that crews had not performed a careful final walk-through with a thermal imaging camera in accordance with North Valley Fire policy.

Further analysis by the department's safety and quality team uncovered reports that crews rarely followed the policy. As a matter of fact, though the policy was known to new fire fighters, several veteran company officers were not aware that the department had implemented the practice of completing a secondary overhaul using a thermal imager. In addition, the company officers from the last units on scene stated that they were extremely tired and were focused on getting their crews rehabilitated and back to the station for some rest and rehydration. More importantly, the safety and quality team found that two of the newer fire fighters (one on Engine 118 and one on Ladder 83) stated they knew they were supposed to perform a secondary overhaul but said nothing when they noticed their company officers preparing to depart from the scene. Their reasoning for not speaking up was that they "thought the officers may have received a different direction from Battalion Chief Olivio."

The original Colony Apartments fire had started with a smoldering cigarette left on a plastic chair on balcony. Few responders ever think that small violation of policy or procedure will ever lead to something more catastrophic. Like a smoldering fire, however, sometime policy violations and the seemingly incidental failure of crew members to speak up can lead to major incidents

Maintaining safety, reliability, and performance within an organization that performs dangerous work in a dynamic environment is very difficult. Leaders of these organizations must choose to remain very vigilant. Such efforts can be time consuming and expensive. Operator in the field will consistently move toward doing what practical, but leaders know that what is practical and easy is not always safe. Maintaining a culture that support crew resource management (CRM), however, requires mindful, careful review of problems and points of conflict.

Experiences in the military, airlines, and some dangerous manufacturing industries have demonstrated that certain behaviors and practices are essential for team leaders to remain vigilant, ensure a safer workplace, and minimize errors. These are known as *high-reliability behaviors*. It is necessary to cover these fundamental behaviors and practices, as they are critical to building an organizational culture that supports open, collaborative communication.

Introduction to High-Reliability Organizations

The term **high-reliability organization (HRO)** has gained significant attention since Karl Weick's and Kathleen M. Sutcliffe's sentinel work *Managing the Unexpected: Resilient Performance in an Age of Uncertainty*, which describes the characteristics of organizations that operate in high-risk environments, yet strive to maintain a learning atmosphere so as to minimize chances for error. (See **FIGURE 9.1**.) Charles Perrow wrote an interesting book titled *Normal Accidents: Living with High-Risk Technologies* in which he postulates that accidents and mistakes are a normal by-product of complex systems and risky operations. Weick's and Sutcliffe's view provides a different context. Their HRO checklist provides a rich series of questions that every organization that wishes to improve performance should ask. Importantly, the critical components that make up an HRO are also those that fit tightly with a just culture and an open communication model, such as crew resource management, which relies on collective situational awareness. Critical HRO components include mindfulness, an inclination towards inquiry and doubt as a means of evaluating and updating standard procedure, attention to the complexities of an emergency incident, commitment to resilience, and a willingness to defer to expertise.

Develop a Habit of Mindfulness

Individual team members need to be mindful of their operations, patterns of behavior, and the skills and abilities of their peers, superiors, and subordinates. Maintaining **mindfulness** is difficult, particularly when teams are subject to repeating the same routines or situations over and over again.

Chapter 3 discussed the Rosenbaum case, where complacent behavior had become the norm, partly because that response system was underequipped to handle the typical volume of calls that it received. In emergency medical services (EMS), the term **frequent flyer** is used to describe those individuals who call 9-1-1 repeatedly, often for what appear to be nonemergency situations. After repeated exposures to the same individual with the same routine complaints at the same time in the middle of the night, emergency responders' thought patterns can become stuck in a rut. This is one circumstance where CRM is valuable. When one person on the team recognizes that he or she is becoming angry or stressed because of frequent calls for service from someone who appears to be abusing the emergency system, it is important for him or her to speak up about his or her feelings. By doing so, the emergency responder calls attention to this distracting element or stressor that can affect team performance. This discussion should be held in a controlled environment, rather than at the incident scene or in a patient care setting.

In Chapter 5, examples were described to illustrate how teams lose situational awareness. Teams can become content with the status quo and never question the risks associated with their day-to-day practices and habits. By challenging routine events and behaviors and questioning how a patient might be distracting the team from taking a fresh look at the reported symptoms, team members can maintain a state of collective situational awareness. They must constantly remind themselves of the dangers associated with complacency. Consider the following case.

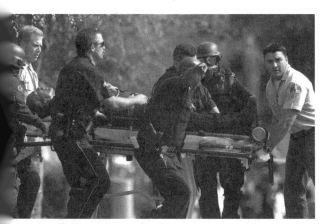

FIGURE 9.1 High-reliability organizations operate in high-risk environments, yet strive to maintain a learning environment so as to minimize the chances for error.

CASE STUDY 2

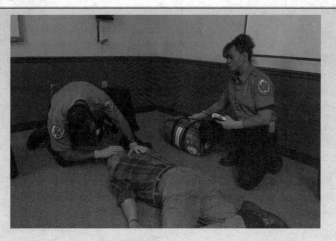

Fire Fighter/Paramedic Jeff Jinks rolled over in bed at the sound of the tones: "Rescue 61, respond to a diabetic problem, 1616 South Twenty-Sixth Avenue, Apartment 9." "Jesse again!" Jinks yelled, to no one in particular.

He and partner Stacey Wendall, also a fire fighter/paramedic, rolled to the address and discussed Jesse Reldman, whom they had seen nearly every night for the previous month. "Why won't he eat like he's supposed to?" Wendall asked. As they pulled up, they noted that the ambulance had not yet arrived. They walked into Jesse's apartment on the second floor. Ignoring the fact that the apartment looked in disarray, which was unusual, both approached Jesse, who laid on the living room floor fighting attempts by his girlfriend to hold him down. The girlfriend told Wendall and Jinks that Jesse had eaten a late dinner after coming home from work and was watching TV when he suddenly rolled onto the floor, screamed out in pain, and started babbling incoherently. When she tried to keep him from crashing into a nearby table, he became mildly combative.

Certain that Jesse was having yet another hypoglycemic reaction ("He always takes too much insulin and forgets to eat," Jinks said later), the two medics started an intravenous line with some difficulty and administered 50 g of dextrose. As they finished administering the medication, Jesse suddenly became unresponsive and held his arms out rigidly. The medics noted that his eyes were deviated to the right, and that it looked like he was having a seizure.

Before Jinks could grab the airway box, Jesse went limp and Wendall noticed that he was now in cardiac and respiratory arrest. They began resuscitation efforts, and Jesse was transported to a nearby hospital where he was diagnosed as having an intracranial bleed caused by a ruptured aneurysm.

During a postincident analysis, Jinks and Wendall understood that although the administration of dextrose was inappropriate in this particular case, there really was nothing they could have done to save Jesse from the catastrophic injury that he suffered. Just the same, this incident is a powerful reminder of how easy it is to become complacent, and how decisions are affected by those patterns that are seen day after day. If Jinks an[d] Wendall wanted to be more effective, if they wanted t[o] embrace and use CRM concepts to help them mainta[in] situational awareness, they would have discussed a[ny] possible performance-shaping factors while en rou[te] to the incident. An example of a successful approac[h] follows.

CASE STUDY 3

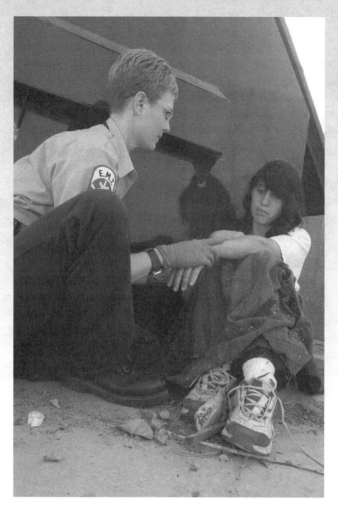

Engine 20 heard the speakers "go live" at the same moment the lights started to slowly come up. It was 2:00 AM, and all four crew members heard the dispatcher announce an address they were extremely familiar with. "Engine 20, code 3, 6767 Sage Drive, apartment number 56, on a patient with shortness of breath." Engine 20 had been to this address, home of Julie Rider, nine times in the previous two weeks. Julie had an anxiety disorder, and everyone on the crew knew what to expect: They would have to sit and calm Julie down; she would refuse transport (along with her medications); and another hour of their life would be spent helping someone who refused to manage her own medical problems.

As they drove to the address, Captain Thaler listened to his crew complain over the intercom. "Why can't she take her meds?" "Let's help her move to Engine 31's first due area." Thaler then recalled his recent CRM refresher training, where his team was asked how they would maintain awareness for risk during routine, day-to-day events. His team had determined that they needed to openly discuss any issues that may affect their performance, including fatigue, distractions, and the simple habitual things they all did while working an incident.

(continues)

> Captain Thaler recognized that his crew on Engine 20, himself included, had become biased about what they would see when they arrived at Julie's residence. So, he spoke up, saying to his crew, "You know, I'm tired of going to Julie's house as well. It's frustrating that she won't care for herself and that she appears to use the system to her advantage. However, I think it's important that we work her up like any other respiratory distress patient. It's good experience, it will help keep us sharp, and we may learn something. We all need to be aware of how our feelings toward Julie have affected our judgment, and how these feelings have closed our minds to any other medical alternatives."
>
> Thaler's crew responded positively, commenting that they were glad someone had mentioned the risks involved. Although they still were not happy about having to respond to Julie's house at 2 o'clock in the morning and, in fact, Julie was having yet another anxiety attack, the example had been set: The crew of Engine 20 was less likely to make a mistake associated with bias and complacency because of this experience.

To evaluate team mindfulness, leaders should ask some of these key questions:
- Is there a sense that the team, or organization, is susceptible to the unexpected?
- Does everyone feel accountable for their actions, and do they value quality?
- Does the team understand what can go wrong, and how?

The only way to evaluate these attributes is to regularly pose the questions.

Avoid Mindlessness

Mindlessness is the absence of mindfulness. It is one's susceptibility to falling into a routine and not paying attention to the small cues that accumulate over time into one major incident. Teams invested in maintaining high reliability guard against mindless behavior by looking carefully at and addressing situations that could foster complacency.

CASE STUDY 4

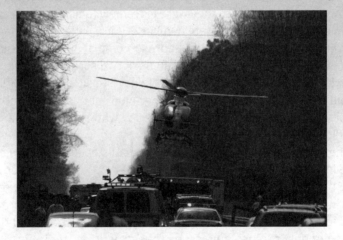

> As Flight Paramedic Jon climbed into the rescue helicopter for the flight to the Clackamas River, the pilot, Charlie, performed the final checks prior to takeoff. In this flight program, the pilots were never told the type of incident the aircraft had been requested for; they only knew the location, which removed

> them from any emotional assessment on whether they should fly. Sue, the flight nurse, and Jon both knew only that they were responding to a traumatic head injury near the upper rapids at McIver Park.
>
> It was a beautiful July day, and the Clackamas River sparkled in the bright sunlight. Hundreds of cars below lined the highway to the recreational areas on Mt. Hood. As the aircraft approached on final, Charlie circled the landing zone and all crew members looked for obstructions and hazards. Seeing none, Charlie flared for landing in a rocky area next to the river.
>
> Before Jon and Sue popped open the doors, Charlie gave his usual reminder, "Stay safe and stay alert!" Jon unplugged his helmet and followed Sue, thinking, "Hey, I love Charlie, but I've been on over 600 flights. You'd think he would dispose of the warning by now."
>
> Moments later, as Jon and Sue departed the aircraft and started walking toward the medical team caring for the patient, Jon noticed an unusually loud, high-pitched whistling sound above his head. As he looked up, he immediately grabbed Sue and motioned upward. They had narrowly avoided walking into the main rotor blades. Because the blades were normally several feet above their heads, both were used to walking nearly upright away from the aircraft. However, the landing zone was next to the river bank, and the ground sloped upward away from the aircraft. In this case, the rotor tips were now only about 6 ft (1.8 m) above the ground on the left side of the helicopter. Jon and Sue posted a fire fighter to guard the area, and they ensured that they approached from the right side when they loaded the patient.
>
> When the helicopter returned to base, Jon told Charlie about his thoughts—how he had been critical of Charlie's usual warning, and then he came face-to-face with a real-life example of mindlessness and habit. Charlie, ever the teacher, kindly held up his metal "kneeboard" used to write down information during a flight. On the back, in large black letters was printed "Don't do anything stupid." He said that he looked at this prior to every flight because you never know when you will do something mindless.

When people are expected to perform their jobs in a particular manner without deviation, when they work under severe time pressure, or when they are tired, they have a tendency to become mindless and operate as if by remote control. This is a serious factor that promotes the loss of situational awareness and leads to many accidents and errors. It is especially important for team members, particularly the team leader, to recognize these types of situations and to draw the team's attention to them. When Charlie constantly reminded his crew to "stay safe and stay alert," he was providing a warning against mindless behavior.

Good teams identify characteristics of a situation that can lead to mindlessness, and they institutionalize methods to ensure that team members remember how to avoid mindlessness during critical operations.

Assess the Ability to Inquire, Doubt, and Update

If any specific pieces of CRM can serve as keystones, they are the parts of the communication loop that provide team members the ability to inquire, express doubt or concern, and update the team on whether the current plan is working.

The Ability to Inquire

Good team environments foster the type of culture where individuals feel free to inquire about what is going on and why. More importantly, team members are allowed and encouraged to check their assumptions about an outcome or process against reality: Is the plan sufficient to accomplish the task at hand? Do the team members have the necessary training and experience to engage at the desired level? Has everyone been informed of the potential dangers? Inquiry, as has been discussed in previous chapters, is often stifled by organizational hierarchy or a culture that discourages people from questioning a procedure, particularly if the organization, or leader, has invested time, money, or expertise in the development of the plan, process, or procedure.

To help encourage the right types of input, leaders should assess whether they are receiving inquiries that challenge the norm. If this rarely occurs, leaders typically assume that their workforce believes in the mission and the way operations are conducted, when in fact team members might recognize serious deficiencies but are reluctant to inquire for fear of retribution.

The Ability to Doubt

In a team setting, it is unfortunately common for members to silently watch someone deny that a problem exists when its existence is evident to everyone else in attendance. Expressing concerns or doubts is a necessary component of healthy, effective team communication. Although it can create conflict, it also allows everyone to be collectively aware of a potential or real problem.

Unfortunately, when team leaders perceive that the existence of a problem will reflect badly on them, many organizational leaders fall into the cognitive dissonance trap discussed earlier. Somehow, they must ignore or deny the problem or ensure that no serious postincident analysis takes place because to analyze the incident would target those in charge.

Creating a culture that allows people to openly question the reason behind actions, decisions, and behaviors is critically important to successful CRM. Many leaders untrained in CRM might look upon this questioning type of behavior by team members as insubordination, but it is a necessary part of creating shared situational analysis. Employees and team members can be taught to deal with conflict and to pose questions in a respectful manner.

Additionally, team members must trust the leader and the leader's motives. This means that stonewalling by the leader won't work because it builds distrust. However, there are times when leaders may not be able to share all information with the team because of legal, competitive, or personal reasons. If that's the case, leaders must openly state that they can't share all the information that was used to arrive at a particular decision. If the culture is one of trust, and the leader doesn't overuse the secrecy excuse, team members generally will accept the leader's decisions, even if those decisions are not completely congruent with their own views.

Some team members may find it difficult to abide by certain decisions when they are focused on micro-issues (immediate details that need to be addressed) and the leader is focused on macro-issues (long-term effects of the decision or larger concepts). Again, these types of conflicts are best managed by the leader openly stating the reasons behind a particular decision and asking team members to provide input continually, particularly if they see things that aren't going well.

HRO performance is directly tied to open communication without reservation. This doesn't mean people can't or shouldn't be respectful and empathetic when expressing doubts, and those who speak up must also understand that their perspective is but one of many. Individuals hold dear their own perceptions and beliefs, but team members may not share these opinions, regardless of how clear the answer appears to a certain individual.

Additionally, leaders must remember that operators—those in the trenches and on the front lines of production and response—truly understand where organizational strengths and weaknesses lie. To operate as an HRO, leaders must encourage these people to express doubt about operations when they have concerns. When a distinct lack of doubt expressed by operators occurs, the organization probably has fostered an environment that discourages feedback.

The Ability to Update

Updating is another key behavior important to the successful use of CRM. A shared understanding of the situation is impossible if team members don't regularly provide updates about their individual perceptions and performance. The failure to update is akin to the failure of a team member to speak up when he perceives a problem with the plan that is presented by the leader.

CASE STUDY 5

Probationary Fire Fighter Renwall followed his partner, Fire Fighter Gitts, closely down the apartment hallway as they searched for fire victims. Visibility was near zero, and all Renwall could make out were the boots of

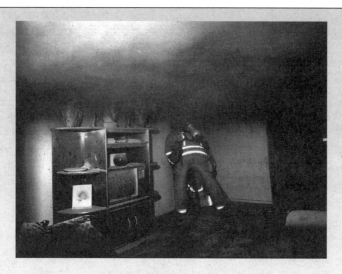

his veteran co-worker ahead of him. Gitts suddenly stopped, and Renwall crawled up next to him, where he could see that two doorways led off the main hallway. Gitts signaled for Renwall to search the room on the left, and Gitts would go right.

As Renwall crawled through the room, sweeping under furniture and feeling on top of the mattress, a piece of sheetrock fell in front of him as the heat level abruptly increased. Renwall grew concerned, and crawled toward the door, peering out to see if the veteran Gitts was finished. He could hear Gitts sweeping through the room, but could not see him. As Renwall considered what to do, the heat started to become unbearable. His neck felt very hot, his turnout coat burned him as he pulled himself close to the floor, and he wondered if he should finish searching the room or call out to Gitts.

While he waited near the door to the bedroom, a large body of fire pushed down out of the room's ceiling, forcing him into the hallway. To keep from getting burned, he moved into the room Gitts was searching, bumping into him. Gitts turned around, pulled close to Renwall, and yelled through his mask, "What's the matter?" Renwall yelled back that the opposite room was being overrun with fire. As Gitts led the way to the door, it was evident to him that the two fire fighters could no longer exit through the hallway. Fire had now flashed overhead and was rolling into the room where they both lay close to the floor.

Gitts slammed the bedroom door closed, grabbed Renwall, and pulled him toward a window that he knew was there from his earlier search. As he called a "mayday" on his radio, he cleared the window frame of debris and pushed Renwall through the opening, where he fell two stories to the ground. Gitts followed, and both were transported to the hospital for burns and traumatic injuries.

During the postincident analysis, this department, which had instituted CRM practices, inquired why Fire fighter Renwall didn't speak up. This was clearly a failure to update, a failure to let other team members know critical information that was necessary for a collective situational awareness. In the CRM loop, updating typically takes place during the observe and critique phase. (See **FIGURE 9.2**.) These critiques are often in fact updates, in which team members provide input related to their specific assignment or their observations.

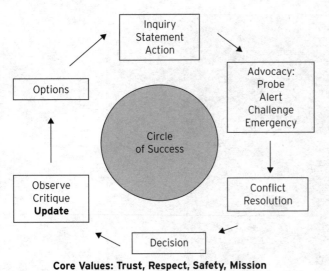

FIGURE 9.2 Updating involves sharing critical information that is necessary for collective situational awareness. In the CRM loop, this takes place during the "Observe and Critique" phase.

around them so that everyone is aware of why a particular decision is being made. However, if another team member sees the environment differently or witnesses a change that could affect operations, it is imperative that the individual speaks up and is heard.

Become Preoccupied with Failure

Being preoccupied with failure seems to be an exercise in futility. Why focus on failure? Why not celebrate success instead?

A focus on failure is important for HROs because they instinctively know that success might be the result of luck, or of a well-developed process or procedure, or because the failure points of the outwardly successful incident have not yet been identified. When a failure occurs, they know something didn't work out as intended. Earlier it was discussed how repeated operations that have successful outcomes can embed themselves in responders' psyches to the point that they believe that every time a particular operation takes place there will be a positive outcome. Members of HROs know this is not the case.

Every PIA, regardless of the incident outcome, provides teams with the opportunity to learn valuable lessons. Sustaining the HRO culture and practicing a commitment to the PIA process are critical for maintaining HRO beliefs within an organization. During a debriefing, what an individual team member may see as a positive outcome may not be so for other team members or for the organization. Leaders must interpret and filter information shared at the PIA, however, ensuring that no facts about the incident or observations by on-scene personnel are "white-washed," or disregarded. Consider the following scenario.

Renwall stated that he knew that he should have said something, but that he was intimidated by Gitts's experience and also wondered whether the heat level was normal. The last thing he wanted was for the veteran Gitts to see him as weak and unable to conduct a search under rough conditions.

Updating, evaluating performance, and critiquing are necessary for all members of the HRO to have a conscious understanding of the entire situation. Every individual has his or her own context, and that context is rich with stimuli. These stimuli are either related to the event at hand or to a similar event that occurred in the past. Processing stimuli in relation to past events is part of the decision-making process discussed in Chapter 4 called recognition-primed decision making. Veterans who operate in this mode often have to update those

CASE STUDY 6

Flight Paramedic Pete Larsen hurriedly prepared the BK-117 helicopter for transporting two patients. This involved removing several pieces of equipment that were stored against the starboard bulkhead and resecuring them in different locations. He had been trained to never remove items from the helicopter and place them on the ground, but instead to leave them in full view on the floor of the aircraft until they were resecured so that nothing critical was left behind. However, since his training had occurred, Pete had more than 200 flights under his belt and the flight program had added several pieces of equipment. As a matter of fact, the pilots routinely complained about the extra weight, threatening to start tossing stuff off.

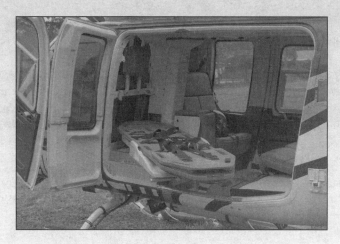

To keep the jumble on the floor from becoming too cumbersome, Pete removed several pieces of equipment and placed them on the port-side skid of the aircraft. He then moved everything around, placed the second stretcher in position, and resecured the items on the floor.

There was the typical muddle of bodies and equipment as both patients were loaded and Pete took a rear-facing position in front of his assigned patient. The nurse, Barb, sat to his immediate left. As the BK lifted off from the accident scene, the helicopter slowly turned left and headed back to Portland. Suddenly, there was a loud banging noise coming from the outside of the aircraft on the port side. The pilot slowed the aircraft and leveled off as the crew members nervously discussed what could be wrong.

Rather than continue, the pilot elected to land nearby so that Pete could get out and look for the source of the problem. He set the aircraft down at the far end of a Target parking lot. As soon as Pete opened the port sliding door, he found the source of the noise—it was the equipment bag for the infusion pump, which he had left on the side step of the aircraft when reconfiguring it for two patients. The carrying strap had wrapped itself around the end of the step, and the bag had rhythmically banged against the belly of the helicopter.

After pulling the bag in, the crew lifted off again and flew to the trauma center in silence. After dropping the patients and giving their reports, they all met to discuss the situation. Pete knew that had the strap not caught on the step, the bag could have damaged the aircraft with catastrophic results.

Instead of burying the issues, this program prided itself on being an HRO. Pete wrote up the incident as a near-miss, and presented the case to the entire workgroup at their next safety session. In addition, the organization revisited the amount of equipment they were carrying and modified the procedures for reconfiguring the aircraft. After that, everyone took turns practicing a reconfiguration with the helicopter running to simulate an actual event.

A focus on failure means that organizations actively seek out and capture the causal factors of any accident, and they create an environment where nonpunitive near-miss reporting is the norm. Near misses and causal factors are then used to refine the training programs and to create necessary redundancies or checklists that simplify complex operations.

This is a true closed loop–complete loop quality management system. Trends are noted and monitored, frequency and sentinel events are recorded, near misses are correlated with "hits" (accidents and errors), and all are fed back into a collective system where operators are responsible for creating system and educational improvements that minimize recurrence of unwanted events. In addition, HROs carefully evaluate human factors to ensure that the system isn't becoming too complex. Complex systems often force individuals into *practical drift* (discussed later), which is the slow uncoupling of policy and actual procedure.

Be Reluctant to Simplify

It can be tempting to provide simple explanations for complex events. Often, the cause of an accident or incident appears obvious: If only the operator hadn't acted in the way he did, the incident never would have occurred. So, simply, it must be the operator's fault. Correct or replace the operator, and the problem is solved.

It is common to give such simple explanations, but by doing so teams fail to become learning organizations. As described in Chapter 3, creating a learning culture comes from looking deeply into failures in a nonpunitive, comprehensive way. Unfortunately, this takes time and resources—both of which are lacking in many public and private organizations. However, an agency need not analyze every single negative outcome to find nuggets of information that will help it become more reliable and safe. By carefully choosing events, organizations can pick representative incidents to dissect to find systemic and cultural trends that are likely causing many of the mistakes being made. In this manner, organizations can focus their limited resources, carefully deconstruct incidents to categorize causal factors, and minimize any tendency to simplify an explanation.

Additionally, attempts to standardize and simplify complex operational practices can have unwanted consequences. Because the environment of the emergency responder is extremely dynamic, the best field procedures leave room for some operator discretion and interpretation of the incident circumstances. Good field procedures or protocols should provide guidelines, be brief (checklists are great), outline risks, and mention any key issues that operators should consider.

On the other hand, one place where simplification can be helpful is in standardizing equipment. Many EMS and fire providers standardize equipment to reduce operational ambiguity, improve training, and reduce errors related to equipment unfamiliarity as operators move between stations and units. However, when human behavior and complex situations cross paths, even simplifying equipment choices and procedures can have unwanted outcomes, as demonstrated in the following case. The lesson is to consider, in depth, all the pros and cons of any decision to simplify operational procedures or methods.

CASE STUDY 7

Paramedic Alicia Wender pulled her ambulance to a stop in front of the apartment building, deftly swinging around the fire engine parked in the street. Her partner of four months, Paramedic Ed Hughes, looked nervous. He had mentioned while they were en route that this was his first call involving a child in cardiac arrest, and the crew of Engine 9 had told them over the radio that they were on scene with a two-year-old boy who was not breathing.

Walking into the front room was a surreal experience. Two fire fighter/paramedics were performing CPR, the lieutenant was holding the child's mother, and the apparatus operator from Engine 9 was digging through equipment bags. Alicia turned to Ed and told him to get the airway equipment out of their pediatric bag.

Small and black, made from heavy-duty canvas, the pediatric bag held all of the critical equipment needed to resuscitate children. Each of its five zippered compartments were held closed by small, breakable seals, and on each seal was printed a date with initials. These represented the next expiration date of any equipment inside that particular compartment, and the initials were of the last person who checked and secured the equipment.

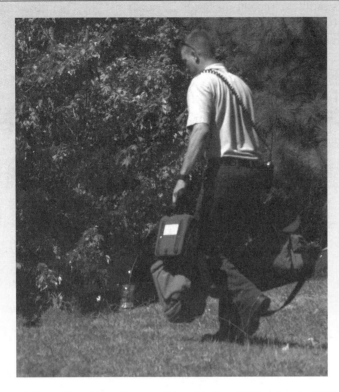

While Alicia assisted the fire medics with the child's airway, Ed broke into the sealed compartments one after another, frantically looking for the airway equipment. Alicia hollered at him to "hurry up, he has a blockage and I need the Magill forceps!" Finally, frustrated and shaking, Ed turned the entire bag upside down and shook all the contents onto the living room floor, digging through everything until he located the necessary equipment.

When the crews were finally ready to transport the child, one of the fire fighters grabbed a biohazard bag and quickly scraped up all the loose pediatric equipment off the floor so that the crews could use it during their trip to the hospital.

After dropping the child off, Alicia and Ed sat down to review the call. Ed, nearly inconsolable because of the incident with the pediatric bag, assumed he would be written up for inappropriate behavior, and worse, he felt completely incompetent. Alicia knew different, and called their EMS chief to meet with the two of them and the crew of fire fighters.

In analyzing the event, it became apparent that this was a system error caused by an attempt to simplify and streamline operations. At some point, someone thought it would save time checking equipment every morning if the agency moved away from the practice of checking each equipment compartment every shift and instead sealed the compartments closed with tabs that indicated when they would need to be opened again (usually for the expiration of drugs or disposable equipment). This caused a situation where individual paramedics might go six months to a year without ever seeing the inside of a particular compartment. In a complex environment, while under pressure, anyone would have difficulty recalling exactly what was in each compartment and where specific equipment was located.

The HRO is reluctant to simplify and looks to correct situations where the organization has created less preincident interaction between critical operators and their equipment. During an incident is no time for team members to be learning how things go together, where they are located, or how they might interact with other procedures and equipment.

Also, organizations that simplify explanations tend to miss the rich learning that is embedded in each event. For example, the most expeditious and common response to an accident or unwanted outcome is to blame the operator. *Pilot error* is a term commonly used by the media. Unfortunately, the true explanation is never really that simple.

CASE STUDY 8

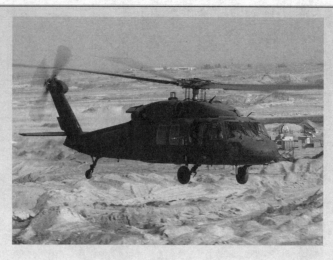

At 8:22 AM on April 14, 1991, shortly after the conclusion of Operation Desert Storm and the Persian Gulf War, two U.S. Army Blackhawk helicopters were flying a humanitarian relief mission inside the "no-fly" zone in northern Iraq. Including crew and passengers, there were a total of 26 people on board both helicopters. A U.S. Air Force AWACS plane arrived on station over the no-fly zone just about 20 minutes after the helicopters departed, and it took a position high overhead where it was to control fighter aircraft entering the no fly zone all day long to keep the airspace clear.

Approximately two hours later, two more U.S. aircraft entered the no fly zone—two Air Force F-15C fighters, which were responsible for "sanitizing" the air space that morning in preparation for all other flights. At that point, there was a total of five aircraft inside the no-fly zone, all American, and all with specific missions and goals.

Shortly after the F-15 fighters entered the airspace, they encountered "hits" on their radar, indicating unknown low-flying aircraft. When the AWACS plane was informed by the F-15s that they had radar contact with low and slow-flying aircraft, it responded in a short communication indicating that it had no specific information related to the potential targets.

Within minutes, the F-15s had identified two enemy "Hind" helicopters, engaged them, and shot them down. Tragically, they were not Hind helicopters, but the two U.S. Army aircraft, and all 26 people aboard were killed instantly.

In reading Scott Snook's detailed synopsis of the incident, *Friendly Fire*, one might first become troubled by the apparent lack of coordination and interagency collective situational awareness. How could there be five U.S. aircraft in the same airspace, where one of them, the AWACS, is specifically charged with monitoring flight operations? How could the two fighter jets shoot down the two helicopters? How tough can it be to figure out whether an aircraft is friend or enemy? It would seem that the AWACS was to blame; after all, its responsibility was to monitor flight operations. But maybe it was the fighters' fault because the U.S. Army helicopters were easily identifiable, each plastered with six American flags measuring approximately 3 feet across by 2 feet high. Who couldn't see that?

Of course it's not that simple. Snook's account is a richly detailed view of how complex systems and operations often interact successfully while no one is aware that there is a slow, inexorable march toward disaster. Only by focusing on its failures does a team come to understand which factors will cause the most difficulty in the future. Snook coins the term **practical drift** to describe how policies and procedure—those written rules we come to rely on for a successful outcome—become background context for most operators, particularly veterans. Agencies that write more rules and policy in reaction to a bad outcome often believe they are solving the problem, when in many cases, they are only creating more layers of dense interacting procedures that will eventually become no more than "BHBs" (big honking binders), destined to sit on a shelf until something falls through the cracks and creates another reason to examine them.

HROs focus on failure because that is where the true learning is—inside daily operations, at the tip of the spear, where teams often trade accuracy for speed.

Be Sensitive to Operations

When it is said that HROs must be sensitive to operations, *operations* refers to those functions that are considered to be front line. Whether this is truly operational, like police street patrols or firefighting teams or whether it is the front line of logistical support makes no difference. The important point is that HROs are sensitive to what is happening at every point where policy meets practice. (See **FIGURE 9.3A** and **FIGURE 9.3B**.)

Organizations often rely heavily on written protocols, procedures, policies, and directives. Although these are important, particularly if the HRO keeps them relevant and up to date, they remain background context to actual operations in the field. If the process is not time-compressed, operators can easily use checklists and algorithms for guidance. These are particularly relevant when the resources are expected to be the same every time, all operators have the same training, and the outcome is clearly defined.

These parameters are rarely in place when the operations are taking place in a highly complex, dynamic, and dangerous environment. In such cases, reactions and procedures that operators "on the street" employ are more than likely third-order controls, as mentioned earlier. That is, operators will more likely use procedures that

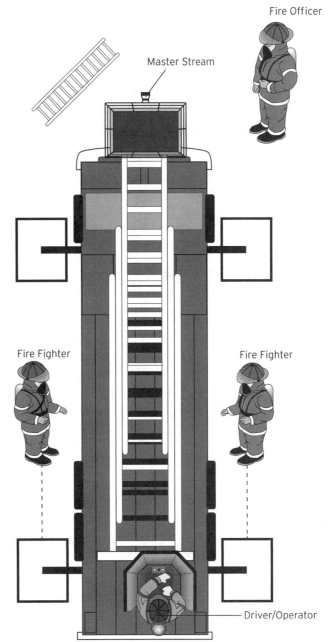

FIGURE 9.3A CRM implementation can ensure the safe and efficient deployment of an aerial master stream from a ladder truck. Each task is assigned and known by each person on the crew. The officer assesses situational awareness, while the driver/operator runs through procedural checks and the establishment of a water supply. Simultaneously, outriggers, ground plates, and safety equipment are deployed by the fire fighters.

align with organizational culture, stories associated with previous outcomes, and repetitive high-fidelity training.

HROs understand that someone with authority and expertise needs to be available at all times during an operational phase (which for many teams is 24/7, 365 days a year). Supervisors need to understand the processes they are responsible for and should be able

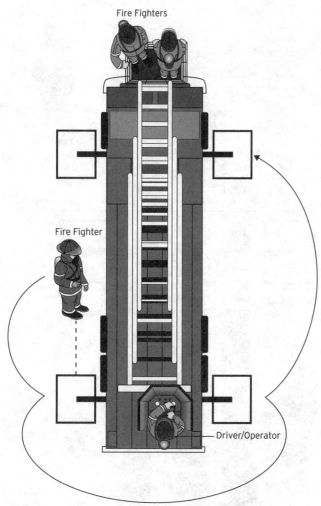

FIGURE 9.3B CRM is easily altered for application in a rescue situation requiring a removal of people by an aerial platform. Key task and mission-specific assignments are designated prior to arrival, and an officer is in place for the assessment of situational awareness.

to pitch in and help whenever necessary. At the same time, they must be sure not to lose overall situational awareness by becoming task-oriented.

The focus on operations is vital when the HRO initiates a systemic cause analysis. During these, organizational hierarchies may be tempted to emphasize the importance of the rules and policies that govern the operations or procedures that are in question. Instead, an HRO drives the process to try to understand where the weak points are to gain a comprehensive picture of how all parts of the operation interact.

Commit to Resilience

By being committed to resilience, an HRO does everything possible to ensure stability during times of turbulence and ambiguity. Ingenuity is important, and the organizational and team flexibility that lead to success come from a commitment to practicing resilient behaviors.

One resilient behavior is instituting, supporting, and continuing high-fidelity training, which is situation-based, hands-on, low-frequency, high-risk-event practice, where teams and individuals are regularly tested under ambiguous and demanding dynamic conditions. This type of training isn't cheap, and it isn't easy to develop. However, it pays big dividends. Flexibility and resilience are necessary if a team's mission is to support people during critical events, particularly when no one involved in the response can guarantee that the infrastructure and resources a team regularly relies on will be intact during a disaster.

HROs try not to run thin in positions where critical skills are needed. They actively work to ensure that teams and individuals have ready access to the resources they need to mitigate events. Teams are encouraged to use their domain expertise in novel and unusual ways to solve problems.

Watching an HRO in action during times of ambiguity and stress is like observing a symphony or a theatrical play. Everyone understands their mission and their role, they know the roles of others, and they are talented enough to cover or improvise when someone misses a cue. Team leaders should think hard about how this applies to their organization, and work to place emphasis on attributes that contribute to resiliency. A commitment to resiliency goes hand in hand with regularly evaluating and updating procedure. In making this commitment, team leaders will prepare their organizations to become industry leaders. (See **FIGURE 9.4**.)

Defer to Expertise

Experts are necessary resources within any HRO. Expertise itself can be overrated, but individuals who have a deep understanding of a particular domain are valuable assets. When the problem is complex, and the technology surrounding it sophisticated, it often takes an expert (or two) to differentiate between those things that a team can ignore and those that are important.

An important attribute for the high-reliability team is a collective understanding related to the power of the team's diversity. Individuals from different backgrounds and experience levels can be richly energized resources when it comes to solving particularly difficult problems. Team members' individual experiences, tied with the team's collective energy and understanding, can be more powerful than a team made up of individuals with similar viewpoints.

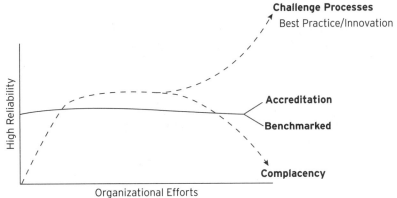

FIGURE 9.4 High-reliability organizations strive to meet a benchmark or accreditation standard. Once that standard is met, an organization often rests on that reputation or achieved standard. Emergency service organizations are dynamic, as is the environment they operate in. It is leadership's duty to continue to challenge the processes to develop best practices or innovation. The validation of these will become the standard or benchmark, thus "raising the bar" for the industry and increasing team reliability.

Deference to expertise is already an ingrained practice within certain high-reliability systems. For example, designated trauma centers, stroke centers, cardiac centers, burn centers, and pediatric centers are all focused on their particular area of expertise. It is well understood, and proven, that the more situations a team member handles within a particular domain, the better he or she becomes at managing those types of critical operations. Individual departments can expand on this concept by developing their own internal strike teams of experts who are ready to engage and solve problems of a particular type.

One example of these expert teams may be the common safety teams that investigate and analyze accidents and incidents. Their domain expertise is usually fairly broad, from documentation to scientific and technical analyses. Another example are teams that are put together to specify equipment. If they involve operators, mechanics, technicians, and supervisors who all have some domain expertise, the result is usually a better outcome.

Leading such a dynamic team can be a challenge. Experts often carry with them a certainty in their methods and a level of confidence built upon repetitive success in their domain. These can be formidable to overcome when conflict arises, and an effective leader keeps the team focused on the mission goals, while allowing creative energy to flow. This requires a conscious understanding of the team dynamics, a personal viewpoint from the leader's perspective that he or she is mainly a facilitator, and the ability to move beyond conflict and use it positively.

Summary

Effective CRM and team communication have demonstrated value in providing a safer environment for both front-line operators and those whom they serve. Organizationally, several factors need attention to provide a highly reliable culture, one that embraces open communication and human error as a basis for continual learning.

Mindful behavior is constant work. No one individual is capable of continual mindfulness, and therein lies one of the critical basic needs for CRM. Only by supporting open communication and a collaborative environment can organizations continually learn from the experiences of all the individuals that make up a team.

Allowing people to question, to ask why, can enlighten the leaders of any organization. These questions, however, can feel like an inquisition or like second-guessing. Leaders should teach team members how to question respectfully and how to resolve and deal with conflict. By building trust, when leaders cannot share all the reasons behind a particular decision in certain situations, they will be able to do so without raising concern among their team.

It can be tempting to anyone who has more responsibility than resources to simplify explanations of error and develop shortcuts for complex tasks. Simplification can also be attractive to those who must answer to policymakers or the media and to people who want to hold someone accountable without truly understanding the complexity of the incident. However, learning doesn't happen through simplification. Learning occurs when teams look deeper for explanations, think hard about the consequences of their decisions, and spend the time needed to ensure procedures have minimal risk to the field operators and their customers. At times, operators must trade accuracy and safety for speed, but those occasions should be in the field, where pure intuition is at work, and not in the after-action analysis of a complex event that resulted in an unwanted outcome.

Focusing on operations must always be a priority if an organization wishes to maintain high reliability and fully utilize CRM as a communication tool. Solutions that are developed in the office do not tend to translate very well to the field. This is where the value of a team really comes into focus. Any team that is chartered to look into operational improvements or changes needs to include front-line operators as key members. Only these individuals can reliably say whether the organizational culture, training, systems, or equipment is up to the task.

Additionally, HROs value the diverse backgrounds and experience levels of their team members. Individual responders will have expertise in unique areas, which is a valuable resource when solving difficult issues. HROs are willing to defer to the expertise of individuals to improve the team's collective energy as well as its understanding of a variety of response situations.

Building highly reliable teams also provides some resilience to the organization in that people are cross-trained in other disciplines and have a broader understanding of the types of issues that affect decision making in the corporate office. Resilient teams respond better to stress, they learn from their mistakes, and they tend to view bad outcomes through a lens that allows personal and organizational forgiveness. Because the errors of front-line fire and medical professionals can have grave consequences, this resilience is important to maintain a positive outlook and culture.

Implementing an open, collaborative communication model like CRM is a difficult job. The task requires top-to-bottom commitment, allocation of resources for high-fidelity training, operator-driven quality improvement, and a leader who is dedicated to high-reliability practices and behaviors. The leader must work with middle managers, unit level commanders, union leaders, and rank-and-file operators to build and embrace a "just culture" environment. The culture must be resilient enough that the organization is able to learn from errors without being punitive. Additionally, the culture must allow individuals to manage negative organizational and personal stories when they are recognized. The organization itself must dedicate regular training and tools on how to manage conflict, and it must work to develop a self-reflective attitude among all members.

None of this can be accomplished through a short class, nor can only one part of the organization commit to making a change. In order to succeed, the principles and practices of crew resource management, team building, and high-reliability organizations must be performed by everyone, at every level, on a continuing basis. CRM opens the door to a heightened level of performance that will provide a safer atmosphere for the front-line operators, a better experience for the end-use customers, and a treasure trove of information that will allow training officers and educators to focus their efforts on the most critical aspects of the job.

Most importantly, when a group works to implement a culture that can effectively use CRM, they are working toward becoming a learning organization. Open, collaborative communication in a safe environment will help maintain a collective force of knowledge and talent, and a team that can overcome nearly any obstacle.

Wrap Up

Ready for Review

- The term high-reliability organization (HRO) describes organizations that operate in high-risk environments, yet strive to maintain a learning atmosphere so as to minimize chances for error.
- Inquiry is often stifled by an organizational hierarchy or culture that discourages people from questioning standard procedure. This is particularly true if an organization or leader has invested his or her time, money, and/or expertise in the development of a plan or process.
- The HRO has a reluctance to simplify and looks to correct situations where the organization has created less preincident interaction between critical operators and their equipment.
- Organizations often heavily rely upon written protocols, procedures, policies, and directives. While these are important, particularly if the HRO regularly updates them to ensure their relevance, policies and procedure should remain only as background context for operations in the field.
- Good team environments will foster a culture in which individuals feel free to inquire about what is going on and why. More importantly, they will allow and encourage team members to assess their assumptions, related to an outcome or process, with respect to the reality of an incident.

Vital Vocabulary

Frequent flyer Those unique individuals who call 9-1-1 repeatedly, often for what appear to be nonemergency situations.

High-reliability organization (HRO) An organization that operates in high-risk environments, yet strive to maintain a learning atmosphere so as to minimize chances for error.

Mindfulness Team members' awareness of their operations, patterns of behavior, and the skills and abilities of their peers, superiors, and subordinates.

Mindlessness The absence of mindfulness; team members' susceptibility to falling into a routine and not paying attention to the small cues that accumulate over time into one major incident.

Practical drift The slow uncoupling of policy and actual procedure. Policies and procedure—those written rules operators come to rely on for a successful outcome—become background context for most operators, particularly veterans.

Assessment in Action

1. Leaders should:
   A. expect blind obedience from followers.
   B. expect followers to question their decisions.
   C. be curious about the problem they are faced with.
   D. Both B and C are correct.
2. High-reliability organizations (HROs):
   A. are rigid organizations that do not tolerate errors.
   B. abide by "just organization" principals.
   C. prefer communication to occur from the top down.
   D. assume that risk is the cost of doing business.
3. A focus on failure includes all but which of the following?
   A. Seeks out and captures the causal factors of any accident.
   B. Creates an environment where nonpunitive near-miss reporting is the norm.
   C. Must be documented to discipline participants.
   D. Near misses and causal factors are used to refine training programs.
4. Practical drift:
   A. causes policy and procedure to become background information for veterans.
   B. causes teams to lose integrity.
   C. only affects the fire service.
   D. is the difference between SOPs and verbal orders.

In-Classroom Activity

Refer students to Case Study 7. Lead a discussion of the issues associated with simplifying procedures and the needs of certain incident locations. Discuss circumstances where simplification of procedures sometimes occurs within emergency response organizations, and what the result is.

References

1. Charles Perrow, *Normal Accidents: Living with High-Risk Technologies* (Princeton, NJ: Princeton University Press, 1999).
2. Karl Weick and Kathleen M. Sutcliffe, *Managing the Unexpected: Resilient Performance in an Age of Uncertainty* (San Francisco, CA: John Wiley & Sons, Inc., 2007).
3. Scott A. Snook, *Friendly Fire: The Accidental Shootdown of U.S. Black Hawks Over Northern Iraq* (Princeton, NJ: Princeton University Press, 2000).

References and Resources

Crew Resource Management and Situational Awareness

Anthony T. Kern, *Controlling Pilot Error: Culture, Environment, and CRM* (New York, NY: The McGraw-Hill Companies, Inc., 2001).
Daniel E. Maurino, et al., *Beyond Aviation Human Factors* (Burlington, VT: Ashgate Publishing Limited, 1999).
Karl E. Weick and Kathleen M. Sutcliffe, *Managing the Unexpected: Resilient Performance in an Age of Uncertainty* (San Francisco, CA: John Wiley & Sons, Inc., 2007).
Paul A. Kraig, *Controlling Pilot Error: Situational Awareness* (New York, NY: The McGraw-Hill Companies, Inc., 2001).
Rhona Flin, Paul O'Connor, and Margaret Crichton, *Safety at the Sharp End: A Guide to Non-Technical Skills* (Burlington, VT: Ashgate Publishing Limited, 2008).

Decision Making

Gary Klein, *Intuition at Work: Why Developing Your Gut Instincts Will Make You Better at What You Do* (New York, NY: Random House, Inc., 2003).
Gary Klein, *Sources of Power: How People Make Decisions* (Cambridge, MA: The MIT Press, 1998).
James Reason, *The Human Contribution* (Burlington, VT: Ashgate Publishing Limited, 2008).
James Suroweicki, *The Wisdom of Crowds* (New York, NY: Random House, Inc., 2005).
Kenneth R. Hammond, *Judgments Under Stress* (New York, NY: Oxford University Press, Inc., 2000).
Malcolm Gladwell, *Blink* (New York, NY: Time Warner Book Group, 2005).

Error Analysis

Anthony T. Kern. *Darker Shades of Blue: The Rogue Pilot* (New York, NY: The McGraw-Hill Companies, Inc., 1999).
Charles Perrow, *Normal Accidents: Living with High-Risk Technologies* (Princeton, NJ: Princeton University Press, 1999).
Colbert King, "The Death of David Rosenbaum," *Washington Post*, February 25, 2006, page A17.
Diane Vaughan, *The Challenger Launch Decision: Risky Technology, Culture, and Deviance at NASA* (Chicago, IL: The University of Chicago Press, 1996).
Dietrich Dörner, *The Logic of Failure: Recognizing and Avoiding Error in Complex Situations* (New York, NY: Perseus Books Group, 1997).
Douglas A. Wiegmann and Scott A. Shappell, *A Human Error Approach to Aviation Accident Analysis: The Human Factors Analysis and Classification System* (Burlington, VT: Ashgate Publishing Limited, 2003).

Edward Tenner, *Why Things Bite Back: Technology and the Revenge of Unintended Consequences* (New York, NY: Random House, Inc., 1996).

Gerd Gigerenzer, *Adaptive Thinking: Rationality in the Real World* (New York, NY: Oxford University Press, 2000).

James Reason, *Human Error* (Cambridge, UK: Cambridge University Press, 1990).

Marilynn M. Rosenthal and Kathleen M. Sutcliffe, *Medical Error: What Do We Know? What Do We Do?* (San Francisco, CA: John Wiley & Sons, Inc., 2002).

Scott A. Snook, *Friendly Fire: The Accidental Shootdown of U.S. Black Hawks Over Northern Iraq* (Princeton, NJ: Princeton University Press, 2000).

Sydney Dekker, *The Field Guide to Understanding Human Error* (Burlington, VT: Ashgate Publishing Limited, 2006).

Communication and Culture

Annette Simmons, *The Story Factor: Secrets of Influence from the Art of Storytelling* (New York, NY: Perseus Books Group, 2006).

Bill Hollis. "Curiosity and Conflict" (Portland, OR: self-published material, 2008).

Carol Tavris, *Mistakes Were Made (But Not by Me): Why We Justify Foolish Beliefs, Bad Decisions, and Hurtful Acts* (Orlando, FL: Harcourt, Inc., 2008).

Daniel Goleman, *Social Intelligence: The New Science of Human Relationships* (New York, NY: Random House, Inc., 2006).

Gerald L. Wilson, *Groups in Context: Leadership & Participation in Small Groups* (New York, NY: The McGraw-Hill Companies, Inc., 2004).

Karl E. Weick, *Sensemaking in Organizations* (Thousand Oaks, CA: Sage Publications, Inc., 1995).

Lee Clarke, *Mission Improbable: Using Fantasy Documents to Tame Disaster* (Chicago, IL: The University of Chicago Press, 1999).

Lee Ross and Richard E. Nisbett, *The Person and the Situation* (New York, NY: The McGraw-Hill Companies, Inc., 1991).

Rhona Flin, *Sitting in the Hot Seat: Leaders and Teams for Critical Incident Management* (Chichester, West Sussex, England: John Wiley & Sons, Inc., 1996).

Robert O. Besco, "To Intervene or Not to Intervene? The Co-Pilot's Catch 22" (white paper, 2004), http://www.crm-devel.org/resources/paper/PACE.PDF.

Sydney Dekker, *Just Culture: Balancing Safety and Accountability* (Burlington, VT: Ashgate Publishing Limited, 2007).

Glossary

Accountability The act of taking responsibility, being answerable and blameworthy for actions taken with the expectation of being called to account.

Air show syndrome Behavioral attributes that are associated with people who need to show off or demonstrate that they are better than others.

Alert When a team member simply and clearly states what he or she is seeing or experiencing that might compromise the mission or objective.

Alienated follower An alienated follower will withhold information due to anger or unresolved conflict with crew members or the leaders and is often looking to sabotage teamwork.

Assertive statement A communication that consists of five parts that enable respectful communication between crew members: (1) an opening statement that uses the addressed person's name, (2) a statement of concern as an owned emotion, (3) a statement of the problem as you see it, (4) the offer of a solution, and (5) obtaining agreement.

Challenge More direct than an alert; when a team member physically moves into the action circle, prepared to take the next step of emergency intervention.

Cognitive control The collection of brain processes that are responsible for planning, cognitive flexibility, abstract thinking, rule acquisition, initiating appropriate actions and inhibiting inappropriate actions, and selecting relevant sensory information.

Cognitive dissonance The state of tension that exists when a person holds or hears ideas, attitudes, or beliefs that are psychologically inconsistent for that person.

Cognitive processing A scientific term for the process of thinking.

Coherence When truth aligns with some specified set of sentences, propositions, or beliefs.

Conflict Actual or perceived opposition of needs, values, and interests.

Conflict resolution A range of processes aimed at alleviating or eliminating sources of conflict; generally includes negotiation, mediation, and diplomacy.

Critical incident stress debriefing (CISD) A confidential peer group discussion in which specially trained teams work with personnel who have been involved in traumatic calls or other painful incidents; CISDs usually occur within 24 to 72 hours of the incident.

Debriefing Allows members who were involved in an incident to speak up in a non-threatening environment, to bring out issues that can be collectively discussed and resolved.

Debunking The process of correcting information about events that have been inaccurately recorded.

Decision point A specific time during an event when an action is selected that influences the outcome of the event.

Dependent individual errors Errors that occur when some of the information available to the operator is incorrect, incomplete, or absent.

Diversity of opinion When people respectfully speak their opinions when they can offer input gained from diverse experiences, domain expertise, and technical operating aptitudes.

Emergency intervention (EI) When a team member takes a direct action to immediately save an individual or the team from harm.

Experiential learning The process of making meaning from direct experience.

Frequent flyer Those unique individuals who call 9-1-1 repeatedly, often for what appear to be nonemergency situations.

High-fidelity training Simulation-based training that often uses real settings or computer simulators and that is designed to help field operators gain recognition-primed experience in low-frequency, high-risk events.

High-reliability organization (HRO) An organization that operates in high-risk environments, yet strives to maintain a learning atmosphere so as to minimize chances for error.

Hot wash A meeting of all responding personnel on a scene to participate in an informal debriefing of the events of the incident, actions taken, and problems encountered.

Humanware The people who are part of a team that has been directed to solve a particular problem.

Incident command system (ICS) A management tool that helps people manage emergency incidents by identifying incident needs and setting priorities.

Independent individual errors Errors that occur when an operator has the correct information but makes a mistake in cognitively processing the information or is "task saturated."

Just culture A culture in which a holistic, systematic approach is taken to understand precisely why an individual or team made the decision or series of decisions that led to what is viewed retrospectively as an undesired outcome.

Line-of-duty death A fatality to an emergency worker that occurs in the course of responding to, training for, or providing service to the public.

Mentor An individual with more experience in the domain, and often older, who helps guide another individual's professional and personal development.

Mindfulness Team members' awareness of their operations, patterns of behavior, and the skills and abilities of their peers, superiors, and subordinates.

Mindlessness The absence of mindfulness; team members' susceptibility to falling into a routine and not paying attention to the small cues that accumulate over time into one major incident.

National Institute for Occupational Safety and Health (NIOSH) U.S. federal agency responsible for research and development on occupational safety and health issues.

National Interagency Incident Management System (NIIMS) A system used to coordinate emergency preparedness and incident management among various federal, state, and local agencies.

Near miss An incident that almost caused a serious accident or injury, but didn't.

Normalization of deviance A long-term phenomenon in which individuals or teams repeatedly accept a lower standard of performance until that standard becomes the norm.

Operators Those on the front line who are engaged in or in command of high-risk operations.

Organizational culture The psychology, attitudes, experiences, beliefs, and values (personal and cultural) of an organization.

Organizational story The texts, spoken or written, as well as visual recollections that usually involve a plot of different interconnected events and bind different characters together.

PACE A method used to challenge team decisions in an assertive and respectful way; Probing, Alerting, Challenging, and taking Emergency Interventions.

PIA facilitator An individual who oversees the process of leading participants through a reconstruction of events, actions, and procedures that occurred during a response to an incident, with the outcome of improving future performance.

Postincident analysis (PIA) An activity involving command and response personnel, taking place after an incident response. It reviews performance of individuals and teams, while focusing on learning lessons that can be applied to future incidents.

Practical drift The slow uncoupling of policy and actual procedure. Policies and procedure—those written rules operators come to rely on for a successful outcome—become background context for most operators, particularly veterans.

Recognition-primed decision Quick, effective decisions that operators make when faced with complex situations. In this model, the decision maker is assumed to generate a possible course of action, compare it to the constraints imposed by the situation, and select the first course of action that is not rejected.

Recognition-primed decision making When a responder *recognizes* a situation based on his or her experience and is *primed* to act in a certain way based on a previous successful (or unsuccessful) outcome.

Rule-based analysis Attempts to capture knowledge of domain experts into expressions that can be evaluated and known as rules. These rules can be compiled into a rule base so that operators can evaluate current working conditions against the rule base and chain rules together until they reach a conclusion.

Sense making The ability or attempt to make sense of an ambiguous situation.

Situational awareness The state of being aware of what is happening to understand how information, events, and a person's actions will affect their goals and objectives, both now and in the near future.

Systemic cause analysis (SCA) A class of problem-solving methods that intend to identify the systemic causes of problems or events.

Task allocation The process of directing specific workers to engage in specific tasks in numbers appropriate to the current situation.

Trend files A database that contains information collected in near-miss accounts.

Veteran's bias When younger team members are influenced to deviate from established practices by veteran crew members.

Wildland/urban interface Geographical areas where populated areas border wildland areas.

Index

Figures and tables are denoted by f and t following the page numbers.

A

Ability to adjust, 98–100
Accountability, 26–27
Accreditation, 143f
Accuracy for speed trade-off, 18
Advocacy, 76–82, 77f, 88–89
Air show syndrome, 109t, 110
Alert phase, 79–80
Alienated followers, 108
Ambiguity, 62
Amygdala, 83f
Anger, 103f, 108
Antiauthority behavior, 109, 109t
Assertive statements, 57
Asymmetrical coherence, 100
Authority, delegation of, 95

B

Barging, 16
Behaviors
    antiauthority, 109, 109t
    expectations, 4
    of followers, 103, 107–108
    hazardous, 108–110, 109t
    impulsive, 109, 109t
    invulnerable, 107–108, 109t
    team, 57–62
Benchmarks, 143f
Bench strength, 101
Biologic response, 103f
Blame, 12–14, 25
Boundaries, 54–57

C

Challenge by team member, 80–82
Chunking feedback, 42–43, 43f
Circle of success, 73–88
    advocacy, 76–82, 77f
    conflict resolution, 82–83, 82–83f
    decision, 83–85, 83f
    inquiry, 74–76, 74f
    "observe and critique," 85–87, 85f
    options, 87–88, 87f
Circumstances beyond operator control, 31
CISDs (Critical incident stress debriefings), 124
Closed loop-complete loop, 137
Cognitive challenges, 18
Cognitive control, 40
Cognitive dissonance, 12–14, 20
Cognitive processing, 59
Coherence, 74–75
Commitment, 96, 105
Communication, 4
    assertive, 105
    open model, 10, 68, 73–74
Complacency, 27–28, 28f, 64
Complex dynamics, 18
Comprehensive approach, 50–54
Concepts of CRM, 47–68, 124f
    boundaries and trust, 54–57
    comprehensive approach, 50–54
    distractions and focus, 65–67
    engagement methods, 57
    shared understanding of, 49–50
    situational awareness, 58–65, 67–68
    team expertise and flexibility, 54
    understanding error, 65
Conflict, 39, 64
Conflict resolution, 82–83, 82–83f, 89, 102
Core values, 77f
Counterexamples of stories, 18
Critical decision process. *See* Decision making
Critical incident stress debriefings (CISDs), 124

Critically thinking followers, 108
Critique conservation, 85–87, 85f, 89
Cue recognition, 41
Cultural awareness, 67–68
Cultural change in organization, 14–18
Culture for learning, 33–34
Culture of fear, 10
Curiosity, 39, 103f

D
Dangerous variables, 18
Deaths in line of duty, 2–3, 4f
Debriefing, 115
Debunking a story, 17–18
Decision making, 37–45
    challenges to, 105
    in circle of success, 83–85, 83f
    complexity of, 39
    key factors in, 40–42
    novices and veterans, 39, 40–41
    recognition-primed, 76
    risks and rewards of, 42–45
    role of conflict in, 39
    rule-based, 40–41
Decision point, 25
Dedication, 96
Delegation of authority, 95
Dependent followers, 108
Dependent individual errors, 65
Deviations from protocols, 27–28
Disclosure, 33
Discussion of options, 87–88
Distractions, 60, 62, 63f, 65–67, 104–105
Diversity in experience of team, 100, 142
Diversity of opinion, 50, 51f
Doubt, 134
Dynamic environment, 18

E
Education and training failures, 31
Emergency intervention (EI), 82
Emergency scenes. *See* Event-driven scenarios
Emotional intelligence decision making, 66, 67f
Emotional response, 103f, 105
Engagement methods, 57
Errors, 25–27, 30
    acceptable rates, 25
    behavioral issues and, 119
    blame, 12–14, 25
    circumstances beyond operators' control, 119
    dependent individual, 65
    education and training deficiencies, 119
    in emergency medical services, 3, 3f
    evaluation, 31
    human factors and, 119
    independent individual, 65
    in a learning culture, 17
    situational awareness and, 65
    system, 119
    taking responsibility for, 29–30f, 30
    team, 65
Event-driven scenarios, 40–42, 40f
Experiential learning, 89
Expertise, deference to, 142–143

F
Failure
    preoccupation with, 136–138
    system failure, 32
    training failure, 31
Fear
    culture of, 10
    of retribution, 17
Feedback
    chunking, 42–43
    respectful, 53–54
Fixation, 62–63
Flexibility of team, 54
Focus, 65–67
Followers, 103–108
    alienated, 108
    behaviors of, 103, 107–108
    critically thinking, 108
    noncritically thinking, 108
Forms for self-reporting, 32
Frequent flyers, 129

G
Glasgow Coma Scale (GCS), 29
Goals and objectives, 94–95
Group-think, 108

H
Hardware, 3, 5f
Hazardous behavior, 108–110
    antidotes to, 109, 109t
Hazing, 10
High-fidelity training, 14, 14f, 44, 66–67, 142
High-reliability organizations (HROs), 127–144, 129f, 143f
Hot wash, 116–118
Human factor influences, 31
Humanware, 3–5, 5f

I
Implementation of CRM, 71–89
Impulsivity, 109, 109t
Inaccurate narratives, 17
Incident command system (ICS), 4
Incident fact sheet, 121, 123f
Incident summary, 31
Incident timeline, 31

Independent individual errors, 65
Information
    ambiguous, 65–66
    load, 65–66
    variety, 65–66
Inquiry, 74–76, 74f, 88, 133–134
Invulnerability, 109–110, 109t

J
Just culture, 16f, 25–27, 33–34

K
Knowledge, skills, and attitudes (KSAs), 92
Knowledge-based process, 40–41
Known unknowns, 15

L
Language, 66
Leadership, 51–54, 85f, 94–102, 94f
Learning culture, 33–34
Lifelong learners, 107
Limitations, individual and team, 97–98
Line-of-duty deaths, 2–3, 4f
Listening skills, 100–101

M
Machismo, 107f, 110
Medication errors, 3
Mentors and mentoring, 101–102
Merton, Robert K., 66
Methods of engagement, 57
Mindfulness, 129–132
Mindlessness, 132–133

N
National Association of EMS Physicians (NAEMSP), 67
National Interagency Incident Management System (NIIMS), 4
National Intitute for Occupational Safety and Health (NIOSH), 3
Near misses, 32, 115
Noncritically thinking followers, 106
Normalization of deviance, 27
Novices
    decision making and, 39, 41
    sense making in situation, 76
    team behaviors and, 57–58

O
Objectives and goals, 94–95
Obligation, 96
"Observe and critique," 85–87, 85f
Operations, 141–142, 141–142f
Operators, 14
Options, 87–88, 87f, 89

Organizational culture, 5f, 8–20. *See also* Organizational stories
Organizational learning, 32
Organizational stories, 8–20
    cognitive dissonance and, 12–14
    managing, 17–18
    mining of, 14–17
    power of, 10, 10f, 12, 14
    writing one's own, 18–20

P
PACE (Probe, Alert, Challenge, Emergency Intervention), 78–83, 78f, 105
    facilitator, 116, 119f
Pattern matching, 41
Perceptions, 66
Perrow, Charles, 129
Physiologic responses, 66, 67f
PIA. *See* Postincident analysis
Pilot error, 140
Postincident analysis (PIA), 30–31, 113–124
    assumptions behind, 116–118
    idiosyncrasies of, 124
    incidents warranting, 118, 118f
    motivations for, 115–116
    standard operating guidelines for, 119–121
    techniques for conducting formal, 118–119
    tools for, 119–121
Practical drift, 138, 141
Pressing, 107f, 110
Probe, 79
Probies. *See* Novices
Procedures, improper, 64
Protocol, deviations from, 27–28

R
Reasoning, 103f
Recognition-primed decisions, 41–42, 67f
Redundancy in task standards, 68
Regression model, 16, 16f
Relationship management, 102
Reliability. *See* High-reliability organizations (HROs)
Resignation, 109t, 110
Resilience, 142
Respect, establishing, 54, 57
Responsibility, 30, 30f, 95
Retribution, fear of, 17
Risk management, 25, 26f. *See also* Decision making
Rule-based analysis, 40–41

S
SCA. *See* Systemic cause analysis
Self-reporting, 32
Self-view, 12
Sense making, 75–76

Sensory input, reducing, 65–67
Shared understanding, 49–50
Simplification, 138–141
Situational awareness
    error and, 65
    instituting within a culture, 67–68
    leadership and, 96
    minimizing loss of, 62–64
    team behaviors and, 58–62
Situational narrative, 31
Software, 3, 5*f*
Standard operating guidelines (SOGs) for PIAs, 119, 120*f*
Storytelling. *See* Organizational stories
System failure, 32
Systemic cause analysis (SCA), 16, 16*f*, 20, 31–32, 142
System influences, 31

T
Tailboard debriefings, 116–118
Task allocation, 3
Task overload, 63
Task standards, 67–68, 67*f*
Team behaviors, 57–62
    challenge by team member, 80–82
    flexibility, 54
    hazardous, 108–110, 109*t*
    novices and veterans, 57–58
    situation awareness and, 58–62
Team building, 54, 107
Time compression, 18
Training. *See also* High-fidelity training
    failures, 31
Trend files, 32, 117, 117*f*
Trust, establishing and losing, 28–32, 54–57

U
Understanding of CRM, 71–89
Unknown unknowns, 15
Updates, 134–136, 136*f*

V
Veterans
    decision making and, 39, 41–42
    expertise of, deference to, 28, 142–143
    team behaviors and, 57–58
Veteran's bias, 28

W
Wildland/urban interface, 3
Worst-case scenario, 27

Y
Yes people, 108

Photo Credits

Procedures
P.1 © AP Photos

Chapter 1
Case Study 1, page 2 © Steven Townsend/Code 3 Images

Chapter 2
Case Study 1, page 9 Courtesy of PAC Tom Sperduto/U.S. Coast Guard; **2.2** © David Hancock/ShutterStock, Inc.; **2.3** Courtesy of Dennis Wetherhold, Jr.; **Case Study 5, page 19** © Mark C. Ide

Chapter 3
Case Study 1, page 23 © Mark C. Ide; **3.1** Courtesy of the USDA Forest Service; **3.2** © Mikael Karlsson/Alamy Images; **Case Study 3, page 30** © Corbis; **3.3** Courtesy of Captain David Jackson, Saginaw Township Fire Department

Chapter 4
Case Study 1, page 38 © oksana perkins/ShutterStock, Inc.; **4.1** © Dan Myers; **Case Study 2, page 44** © Darryl Vest/ShutterStock, Inc.

Chapter 5
Case Study 1, page 48 © Peter Betts/ShutterStock, Inc.; **Case Study 3, page 55** © Ryan Gardner/AP Photos; **Case Study 4, page 56** © Steve Redick; **5.4** © Mark C. Ide; **Case Study 5, page 59** © photobar/ShutterStock, Inc.

Chapter 6
Case Study 1, page 72 Courtesy of Robin Ressler, PA3/U.S. Coast Guard; **Case Study 2, page 75** © Keith D.Cullom; **Case Study 4, page 77** © Jack Dagley/ShutterStock, Inc.; **6.5** © Oguz Aral/ShutterStock, Inc.; **Case Study 6, page 81** © Steve Townsend/Code 3 Images; **Case Study 7, page 84** © Glen E. Ellman; **6.7** © Glen E. Ellman; **Case Study 9, page 88** Courtesy of Captain David Jackson, Saginaw Township Fire Department

Chapter 7
Case Study 1, page 91 Courtesy of NPS; **Case Study 3, page 95** © Colin Archer/AP Photos; **Case Study 4, page 97** © Sylvia Pitcher Photolibrary/Alamy Images; **Case Study 5, page 99** © Dan Myers

Chapter 8
Case Study 1, page 115 © Warren Parsons/ShutterStock, Inc.; **Case Study 3, page 122** © Dariush M./ShutterStock, Inc.

Chapter 9

9.1 © LM Otero/AP Photos; **Case Study 4, page 133** © Jeff Thrower (WebThrower)/ShutterStock, Inc.; **Case Study 5, page 136** © Keith D. Cullom; **Case Study 6, page 138** © Gualberto Becerra/ShutterStock, Inc.; **Case Study 7, page 140** © Michelle Donahue Hillison/ShutterStock, Inc.; **Case Study 8, page 141** Courtesy of Staff Sgt. Suzanne M. Jenkins/U.S. Air Force

Unless otherwise indicated, all photographs and illustrations are under copyright of Jones and Bartlett Publishers, LLC, courtesy of Maryland Institute for Emergency Medical Services Systems, or have been provided by the authors.

NOTES

NOTES

NOTES

NOTES

NOTES